One With Nature

The act of being part of your environment, without harming it.

Written and Illustrated by Wade Geilow

Co-Author Jonacia Geilow

Copyright © 2012 by Wade Geilow
First Edition – April 2012

ISBN
978-1-77097-456-2 (Paperback)
978-1-77097-457-9 (eBook)

All rights reserved.

No part of this publication may be reproduced in any form, or by any means, electronic or mechanical, including photocopying, recording, or any information browsing, storage, or retrieval system, without permission in writing from the publisher.

This is a book of true events, actual persons and places.

Published by:

FriesenPress
Suite 300 – 852 Fort Street
Victoria, BC, Canada V8W 1H8

www.friesenpress.com

Distributed to the trade by The Ingram Book Company

Contents

Dedication	v	Elk	38
Imagine	1	Moose	39
Green Sea Turtle	3	White Tail Deer	41
The Sea of Cortez	5	Mule Deer	42
Spotted Dolphin	6	The Bald Eagle	44
Dorado	8	Snowy Owl	45
The Whale Shark	9	Great Horned Owl	47
Escape	10	The Elusive Wild Turkey	49
Brook Trout	14	Toucan Bird	50
Rainbow Trout	16	Deinonychus	52
Golden Grouper	18	Man the predator	53
Leopard Grouper	18	Lucky Dog	54
The Morey Eel	20	Water World	55
The Guardian Angel	21	Communication with all	56
The Blue Ringed Octopus	24	Karma	57
The Humboldt Squid	25	Insects	58
Sea Lions	26	Self Control	59
The common Dolphin	28	Plants	60
Humpback Whales	31	Book End	61
Sea Lion Octagon	32	About the Author	63
The Mountain Lions	33		
Bears	36		

Dedication

This book is dedicated to my mom and dad for planting my seed and nurturing my growth and every one whom I have loved and that has loved me. Especially my wife Jonacia, without whom this book would not be possible and without her I would be lost.

My wife is my inspiration. It is because of you I write these words. Your strength, confidence, understanding and love have given me the desire to write this book. You have shown me that you can do anything humanly possible. I admire your fortitude for getting things done and your kindness towards all life. Your ability to communicate with it speaks highly of you. You are humble and true, you give of yourself without asking for anything in return. You are my light in the darkness. My soul mate, I look forward to many years of happiness and wonder with you. We will explore the beauty of this life on earth together and with our bond; we will overcome the obstacles life throws our way. Together we will achieve great happiness and love.

Jonacia
I love you.

Special thanks to my Mom, Terri Moss and Deanna Welsh for helping prepare, type and edit this book.

Imagine

Imagine; our solar system is an atom with a Nucleus (the sun). Earth (an electron) other planetary bodies like the Moon, Venus, and Pluto etcetera, are protons and neutrons. This is our solar system, put it with billions of others and we have a Galaxy (a cell) put this Galaxy together with trillions of other Galaxies and you have a universe (a living being).

Our universe is alive. It makes sense to me; Like the Big Bang Theory, it starts from a seed and bursts into an entity, which is born and grows in to adulthood and then dies. One year to it is like a billion years to us, time passes more slowly for a being of this magnitude. Maybe there are other universes and ours is but one of a never-ending number of them. If our universe is a living entity and it lives on a planet in another solar system in another universe, which is also another living entity that would mean that this repetition of life could go on into infinity. One could also imagine that our body is a universe and one atom amongst the trillions has a proton that is like earth and has life on it similar to our planet. This repetition of life could go on and on in either direction creating an infinite number of dimensions for life to exist.

Disclaimer

In this book, I have used real experiences from my life to tell these tales. These are real people, using their real names and real places. I do not need to protect the innocent for they have nothing to hide.

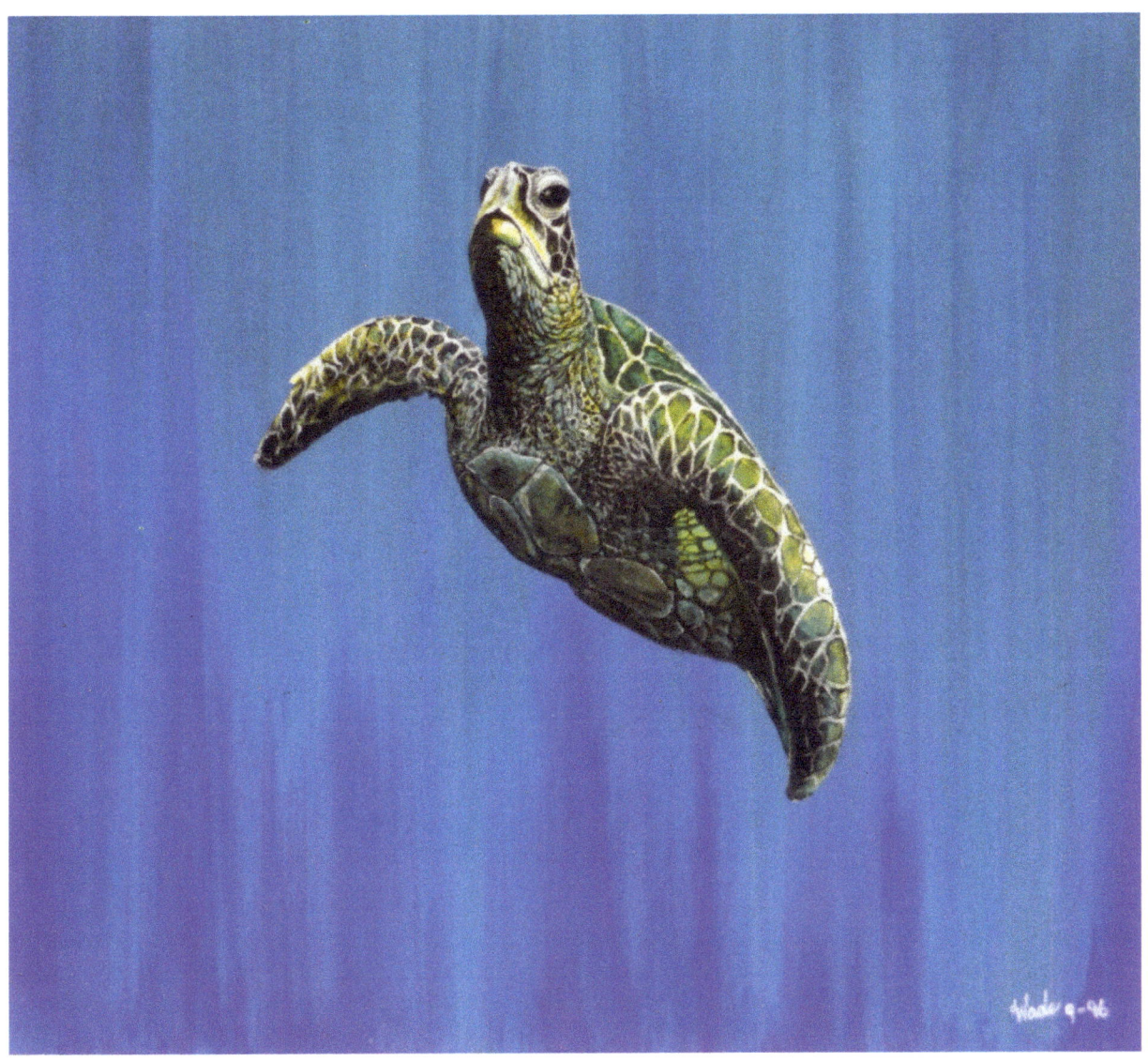

Green Sea Turtle

The green sea turtle is truly one with nature, alone in the sea, in the soup of life.

This graceful creature roams through the great sea, living out its life as part of its environment with out harming it in any

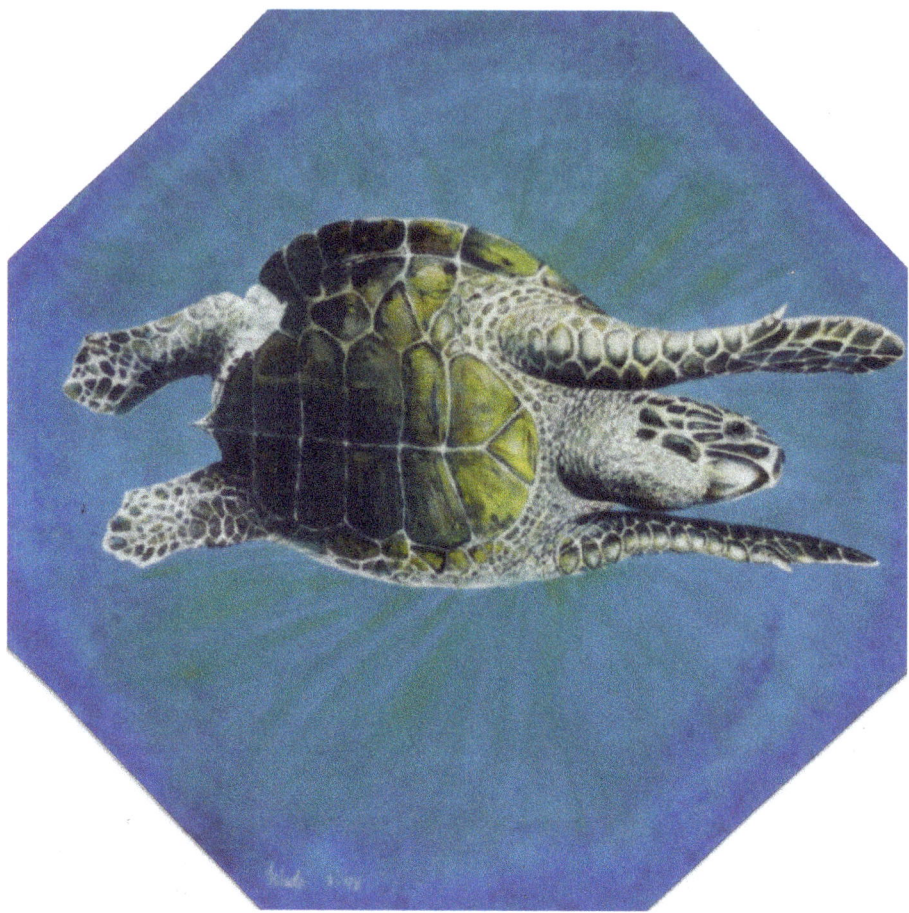

way. An inspiration for many, it is the symbol of this book.

I have only seen one in the wild, in the sea of Cortez (Gulf of California) it was a big one. I was amazed. At first, I thought it was a seal, and then with amazement I realized that it was a turtle. This happened in Bahia De Los Angles "Bay of the Angles, Baja California. This was my first time to visit this wonderful place. I went there with a friend of mine, Kurt and his boss Ken. The boat we went out on, a Boston Whaler, belonged to Ken. This was a perfect fishing boat; it had a center console with dual outboard 150 mercury motors on the transom. It was decked out for fishing, shade from the brutal sun shine, a live bait tank, rod holders, trolling gear and a cooler full of ice cold drinks, there was everything we needed for a great day out, we were set for fishing.

This was the beginning of my adventure, which made me fall in love with the sea and all the creatures in it. I started painting the animals that inspired me. All of which has their own story.

Here before you are some of the paintings of those animals and the tales accompanying them.

The Sea of Cortez

We did the usual boating stuff, water skiing, fishing, swimming, usually close to shore. It depended on how much money we had for gas and what the weather forecast was for the day.

One day Kurt asked me if I would like to go fishing in the sea of Cortez with Ken and his new boat, I jumped at the opportunity. I fell in love with fishing at a young age. My maternal grandfather took me in his canoe on St. Froid Lake in northern Maine where we fished for smelt. He only spoke French but I understood every word he said, at the time. Gramps got me started on a passion that has never left me, that was fishing. This trip with Ken and Kurt was the first of many that would give me experiences most people will never get to experience. For that, I am grateful.

After a long two days of driving, we finally made it there. Ken stopped a lot on the trip to show us the sights and eat, he knew all the good spots to see and all the best restaurants and taco stands to eat at because he had been there many times before.

San Quinton has the best fish taco stand ever, I still to this day cannot duplicate that flavor at any other restaurants or even my self and I fancy myself a good cook.

The sea of Cortez has some of the most beautiful sights I have ever seen. When we drove over the peeks of the mountains, we saw a blue green paradise before us. After hours of driving in a hundred plus temperatures, it was a sight for hot weary eyes. I could not wait to get in that cool refreshing water. My first day out fishing was one of the most wonderful days; I was in awe at getting to see pods of Dolphin, hundreds of them at a time. Ken would slow the boat down when they were swimming next to us so we could get a closer look. We got down on the bow of the boat and pet them as they swam with us; they would look right in our eyes. There was an unspoken communication between the Dolphin and I akin to telepathy. Curiosity, kindness and wonder are what I saw in their eyes. The meeting of an unfamiliar species with no ill intent. I was in heaven "paradise this earth is". The feeling of a bond between the animals and I would continue for the rest of my life. The fishing trip with Ken and Kurt that week was one of the best weeks of my life it changed me forever.

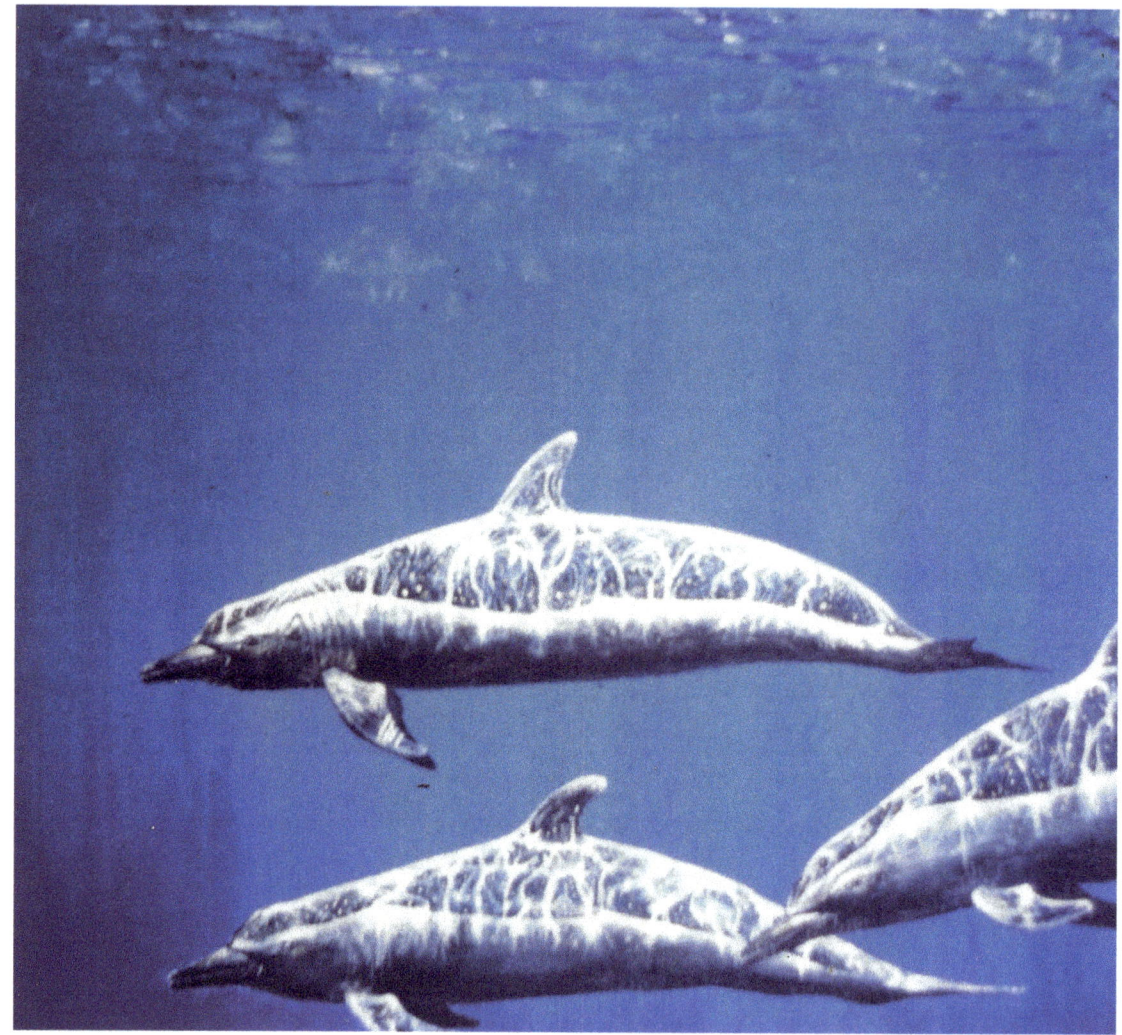

Spotted Dolphin

I recall on the second day we came across a dead whale, probably a grey whale. There were a lot of them at that time in "July". We would see them daily off in the distance surfacing with the usual blow. Getting up close to one like this really gave a true sense of how big they are, at lengths of up to fifty feet and weights of up to thirty-seven tons. I felt bad because this one whale was dead.

Ken proceeded to hook me up with a rod and reel and a metal jig. I had never used this type before, he told me to tie it on and cast out, "The bite is on". Just as he said that, from the cast he just made he hooked up with a Skip Jack tuna. These fish were approximately eight to ten pounds and when they hit the deck, we called them flapjacks. They kept flopping and swimming around on the deck of the boat, which made it a bit dangerous for us because they still had the big metal jigs hanging from there mouths. With Ken's almost instant catch I hurried and tied my jig on then casted out as fast as I could, immediately bird nesting my line. That is when your fishing line bunches up in and around your reel, it was truly a tangled mess and of course I hooked a nice tuna just as it tangled,"wow".

What a tug he put on and twang he was gone, with Ken's new jig. I got my first lesson that day on just how much these jigs cost and how to tie the correct Palomar knot so you do not lose your jig.

For my next lesson, I learned to wear shoes on the boat when fishing, because when I landed the next fish, he was flopping around and I got one of the treble hooks from the jig caught in the heel of my right foot. "Ouch". The fish was flopping (flap jacking) around and so was the hook in my heel "Oh the pain". Therefore, I had to detach the fish as fast as I could to spare myself more agony. After getting the fish off the hook, I asked Ken or Kurt for help in getting the hook out of my foot; well I was on my own. I had to take a pair of needle nosed pliers and drive the barbed part of the hook through the skin and muscle tissue to cut it off, then back the hook out of my heal. Life has its lessons and that was a painful one. With no sympathy, I might add.

This would be the last time I had to remove a hook from myself, "thankfully" it was other people I removed hooks from after that. At least they had help, sympathy and a first aid kit to ease the pain. The day I had to remove my own hook, Ken and Kurt laughed at me the whole time; they were not the nicest guys. They constantly played jokes on each other for fun. Kurt warned me of this on the way down to Bahia. There were a couple of his jokes "pranks" not to fall for. One of Ken's favorites was when driving through the desert on the way to Bahia, he would say something was flapping on the boat and ask you to go check it out and then leave you standing there as he drove off, only to return later laughing at your peril. Then there was the bucket trick. Sometimes when trolling with lures it can get a bit monotonous and tiring, add a few beers and hot sun the person in the fighting chair can easily fall asleep. When that happened Ken would reel in one of the lines, attach a five-gallon bucket to the end of the line and let it back out. Then Ken would put the clicker on and shout "Hook Up" making the sleeping angler jump to attention and start reeling his heart out to get that big catch on deck, well it would be nothing but a bucket. He would keep the boat moving so that the reel would buzz its alarm and the sleepy angler would think he hooked the big one. I found out that you should always check to see if the boat is stopped before reeling like a mad man.

Ken loved a joke and a laugh even at the expense of others. One hot day mid trip, Kurt fell asleep in the fighting chair, unprepared for his battle with the gorilla. Then he hears "Hook Up" he jumped up in excitement grabbing his pole closing the bale, he set the hook and expertly placed himself back in the fighting chair and harnessed himself in for the big fight. He pulled and reeled again and again, the boat is still moving forward under the power of the engine. This goes on for about ten minutes when all of a sudden he realizes he fell for the bucket trick, the one he told me not to fall for. Oh, he was mad, especially when a nice twenty pound Dorado hit my jig while I was holding it in the water next to the boat. Without much effort, I landed the fish and Kurt was livid. "You caught my Dorado", he said. About then he noticed that his line was caught in the propeller shaft of one of the out board motors and he had to jump in and cut it all out. I guess the joke was on him that day. Boy was he mad! After some time I got wise to these tricks and played them on others, all in fun mind you.

Overall, I have seen many wonderful sights, so much life all in one place. Did you know the sea of Cortez has more sea life per square mile than anywhere on earth? I was in awe.

So many birds, mammals and fish, it is hard to believe all this life could live together in one small area. I just had to preserve the memories some how. Out of this came my desire to paint.

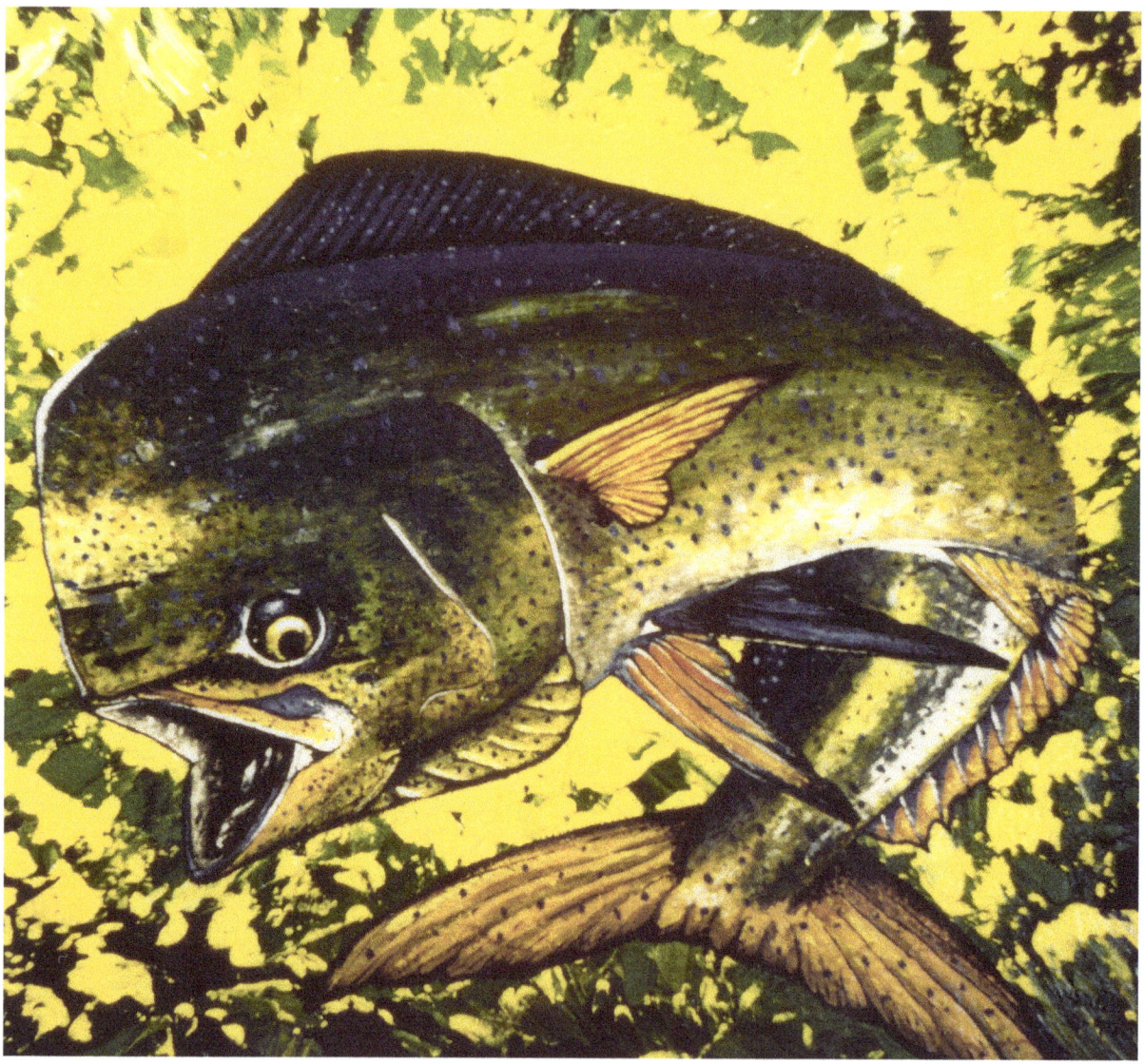

Dorado

This fish is known by three different names, Dorado, Mahi Mahi or Dolphin fish. It is capable of changing its colors from turquoise to green to yellow and then to white sometime sporting all the colors at once. I personally would have to say this is one of the most beautiful of all fish.

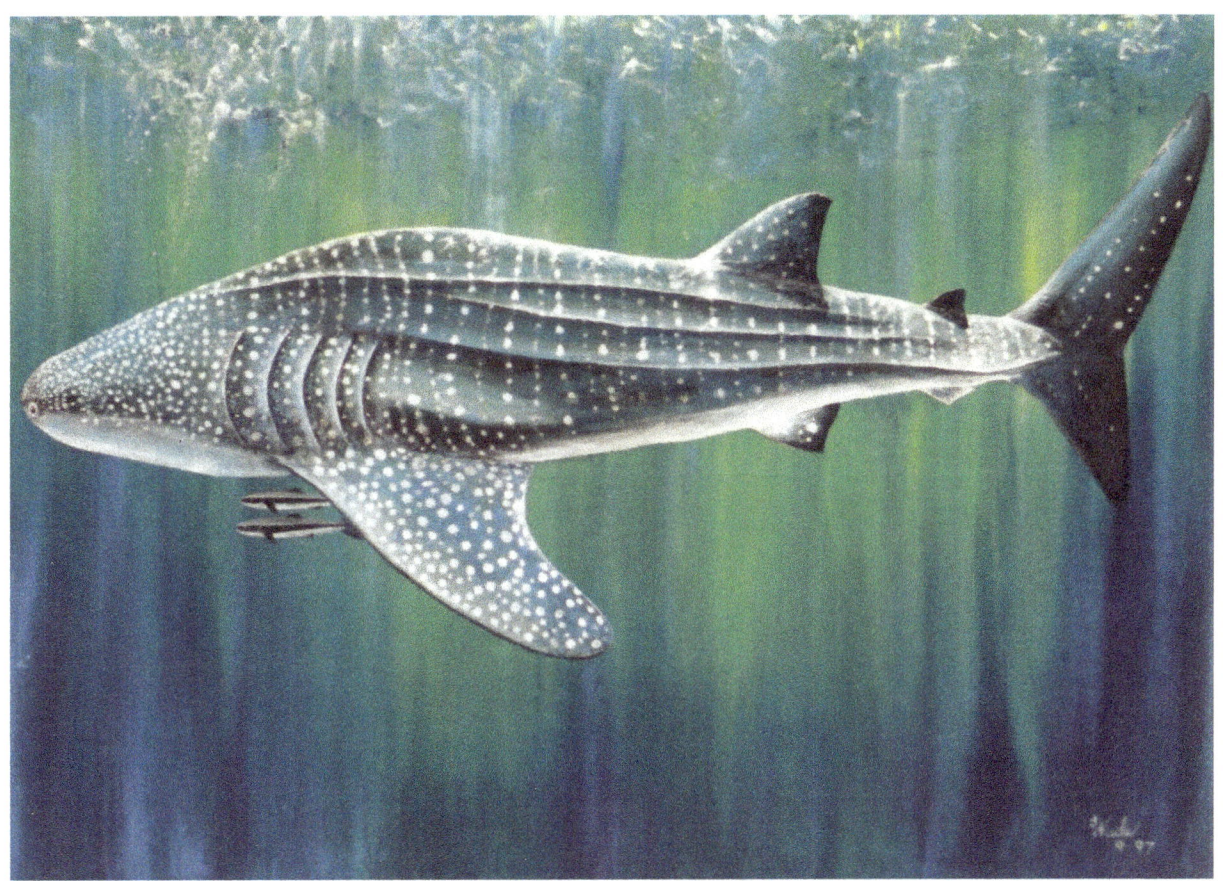

The Whale Shark

Years later on another trip to Bahia De Los Angeles, I was with some friends Russell, Scott and his girl friend; I do not remember her name. After days of getting in our share of fishing, we took a break from it and decided to have a different kind of fun. We were pulling Russell behind the boat on a boogie board in the bay when I spotted a fin sticking out of the water not far behind Russell. "SHARK" I yelled and stopped the boat. My boat was twenty-one foot long, hydra sport, deep V, center console with a 325 Johnson out board motor. It was a fishing machine; it moved like a bullet; and Shotgun was its name. Russell heard shark and I never seen him move so fast. He swam back to the boat and climbed on the boat so fast his hair was still dry. Laughing I put the boat back in motion and went to where I saw the monster, it was a shark all right but not the kind I thought is was, it turned out to be a whale shark about twenty foot long, a baby really. The leviathan swam along with the boat in a way that said come on in. Again that telepathy thing happened and I answered by getting in the water with the giant toddler. I climbed aboard its back and went for the most amazing and memorable ride of my life. It was the coolest thing ever, moving through the warm seawater atop this beautiful, peaceful creature of the deep. I felt as though I was one with the animal and it showed no aggression or fear towards me. It was at peace with me, and its surroundings and I felt the same. I dismounted and left it to its journey in the vast sea it calls home.

Enriched by my experience I asked if anyone else would like to take a ride, much to his or her loss no one else had enough nerve to experience the wonder. There were pictures of this taken by Scott's girl friend, unfortunately she lacked camera skills needed to capture the shot of me on the whale sharks back. What a shame, the closest she got to a story telling photo was a picture of the top of my head, not me on the giants back.

We thought that shark to be huge at twenty foot long. Two days later after Scott and his girlfriend left for the arduous ride home, Russell and I came across one that was at least twice the size of the one I got a ride on. It had to have been forty or more feet long, its head appeared to be eight feet wide, that is not exaggerated, and it looked like it could easily swallow the boat. I am afraid this time I did not have the berries to jump in for that ride. So we just admired in amazement at the calm nature of this animal, its size and beauty and our luck to have gotten this close to such an amazing beast. We took a picture and then left him to his smorgasbord of plankton in the sea of life.

Escape

My friend Kurt, always joking around, a prankster, an angler, a carpenter and many other things I probably should not mention. He was my friend for a long time. We even worked together. Self employed you learn to be tough, so in saying, Kurt was a tough guy, rough voice, talked tough and acted the part. A man of men, nothing scared him, until today. We left in the morning before the sun came up so we could get the early bite on, again ready for our ocean-fishing excursion.

We pulled in to the landing at San Pedro California, just before the dawn light lit the sky. Perfect timing as we headed out to sea looking for sharks. Well we found them. We were out about fifteen miles approximately half way between Catalina Island and San Pedro where the water is deep. From a previous outing, we had a milk crate full of Mackerel we had frozen. Over the top of the crate was wire mesh tide down to create a cage so the sharks could not get at the Mackerel. We poked holes in the Mackerel to create a chum line, or slick,

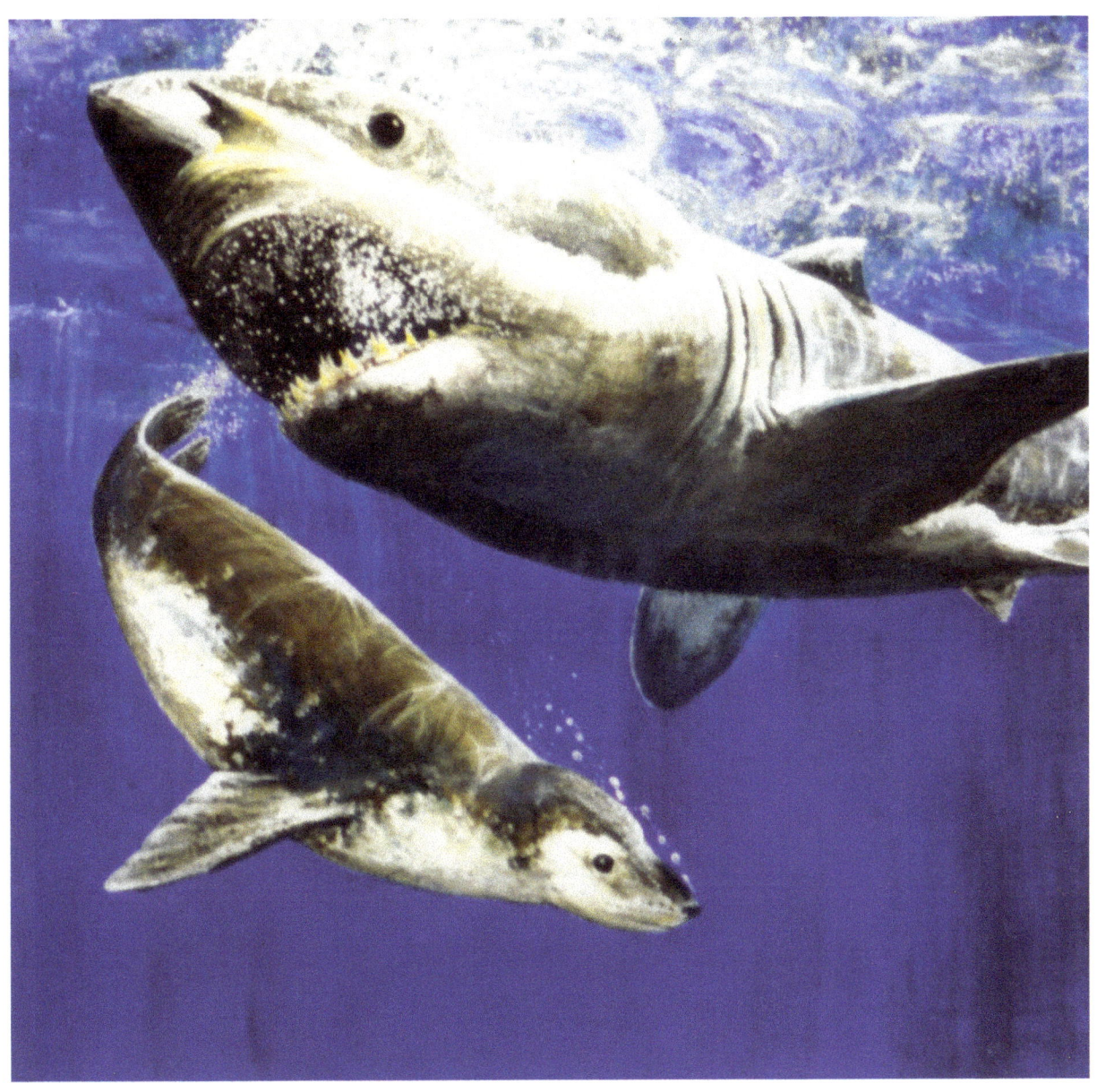

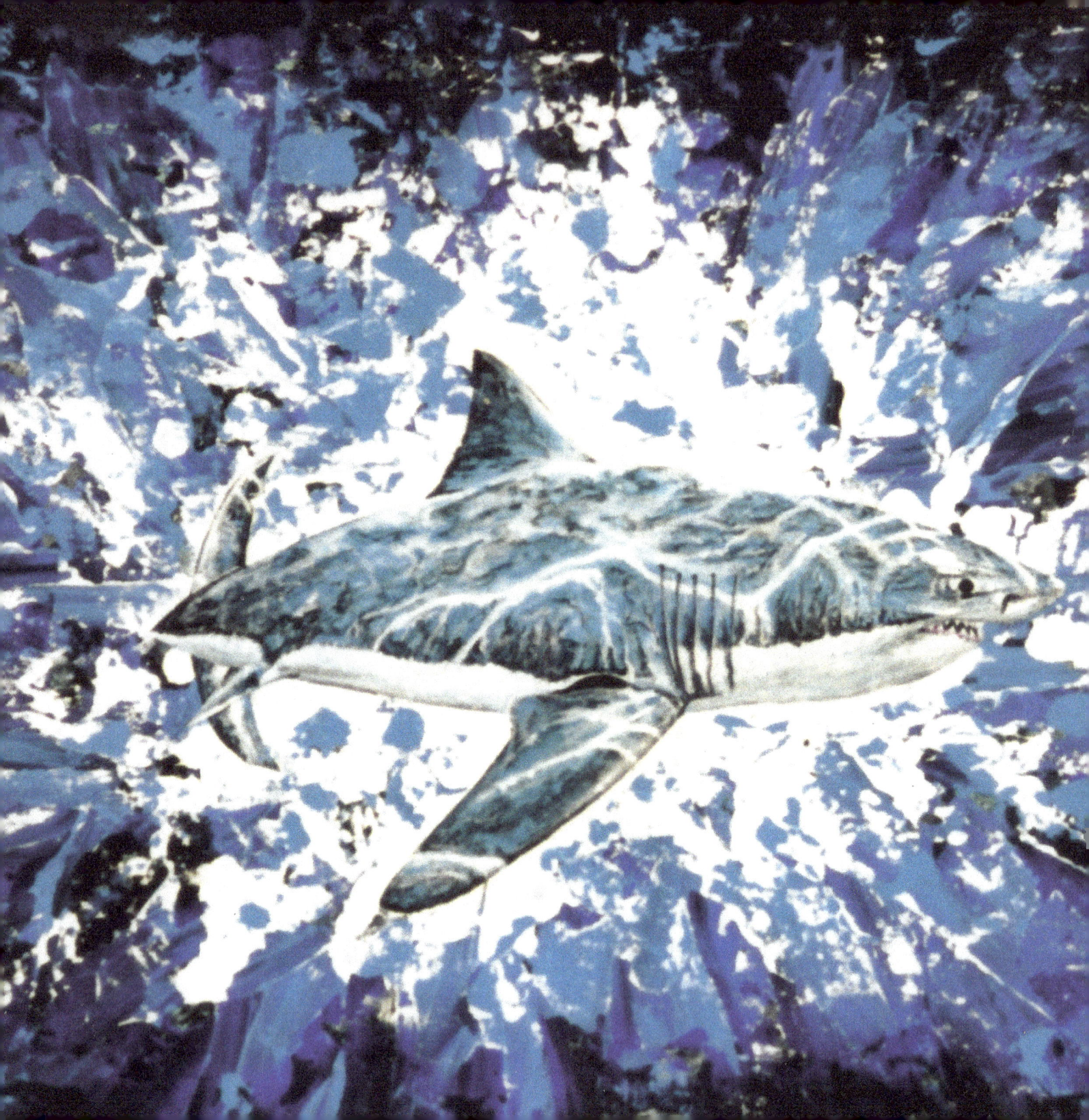

to attract the sharks. I tied one end of a sixteen-foot rope to the crate and the other end to a dog on the back of the boat. No the dog is not rover, a dog is a bracket used for tying the boat to the dock, or in this case chum to the boat. Mind you if something big were to take this chum basket for a picnic it could sink the boat. Of course, if this were to happen we would be floating munchies for these beasts. We could be a much bigger snack for their lunches then those little appetizers in the basket. Boy, we put a lot of thought in that one.

Well, we proceeded to fish with no steel leaders because after all it was catch and release. We had no intension of keeping any thing we caught, so we just used a single hook tied to monofilament line, for the fun and challenge of it. Before we knew it, we had more than a dozen three to six foot blue sharks circling Kurt's boat. Needless to say, we were constantly hooked up for about two hours. We were using light line from forty to fifteen-pound test on the different rod and reels. It was awesome, every time you hooked up and your reel started to sing, as line peeled off the reel, you knew you were in for a fight. We landed maybe fifteen sharks and then suddenly the sharks just disappeared, we were dumbfounded.

After so much excitement, we sat quietly bobbing up and down in the Pacific, boredom started to set in. This went on and on for what seemed like hours but was probably only minutes. Then finally, a click from one of the reels then another click click, then it buzzed as the line peeled off the reel. It was the fifteen-pound set up, the lightest of all the rigs. I grabbed the rod, closed the bale and with a healthy tug I set the hook. My rod bent to the max and I could tell it was something big. I thought the fight was on, but then nothing; it was as if I lost the fish. I started reeling and reeling and then I saw it, a shark coming towards the boat.

Not just any shark, this shark was a Great White. As it approached, I saw my hook hanging off its lip just out side those big teeth. It had its mouth open just enough to see its pearly whites. It was approximately two feet wide at the head and sixteen foot in length, that was as long as the boat. My kneecaps began to shake. As it went under the boat I looked into its big black eye, which was about the size of a fifty-cent piece I suddenly had visions of me being its dinner. I realized my rod was bent to the point of braking when my line snapped with a pop. I then crossed to the other side of the boat in time to watch the shark swim away, so I thought. Meanwhile Kurt was screaming in a high-pitched voice like an eight-year-old schoolgirl, "Jaws, Jaws, pump the ball, pump the ball".

That is all he could say and he kept repeating it as he turned the key trying to start the motor. Ignoring his cries I watched the shark as it turned and headed for the chum box. In fear of the shark grabbing the box I stepped to the transom, grabbed the rope, and started pulling it up. This acted like a lure and the shark picked up speed as if to catch its retreating prey. I kicked myself into survival mode as adrenalin surged through my veins. I pulled on the rope hand over hand until the box was within my reach, as I grabbed the box I fell back and the box landed on my chest.

With legs spread eagle, one foot was on the motor while the other was on the port side of the boat. I pushed the chum box off to see the sharks head on the transom with mouth agape in one last attempt for an easy meal. The shark slipped back into the water unsatisfied with its unsuccessful attempt at the picnic basket. Kurt still squealing like a girl to pump the ball, I reached over and squeezed the ball in the fuel line to prime the motor and just like that, I heard the sound of our escape starting up. Kurt put it in to gear and hit the gas. As we were picking up speed, the shark followed us until we hit full throttle and planed out. Finely we were able to lose it after about a quarter mile. My knees were still shaking and I guess my voice had picked up a notch or two in pitch according to Kurt.

We looked at each other and laughed in relief, because as we were discussing it we realized how close we had come to being lunch for that shark. Because the boat we were in would have easily sunk had the shark taken hold of that chum box and swam with it. In my appreciation for escaping becoming his meal for that day, I painted Escape, which to this day I believe to be my best work. See what a little excitement can do.

This insatiable ruler of the depths is the Great White Shark.

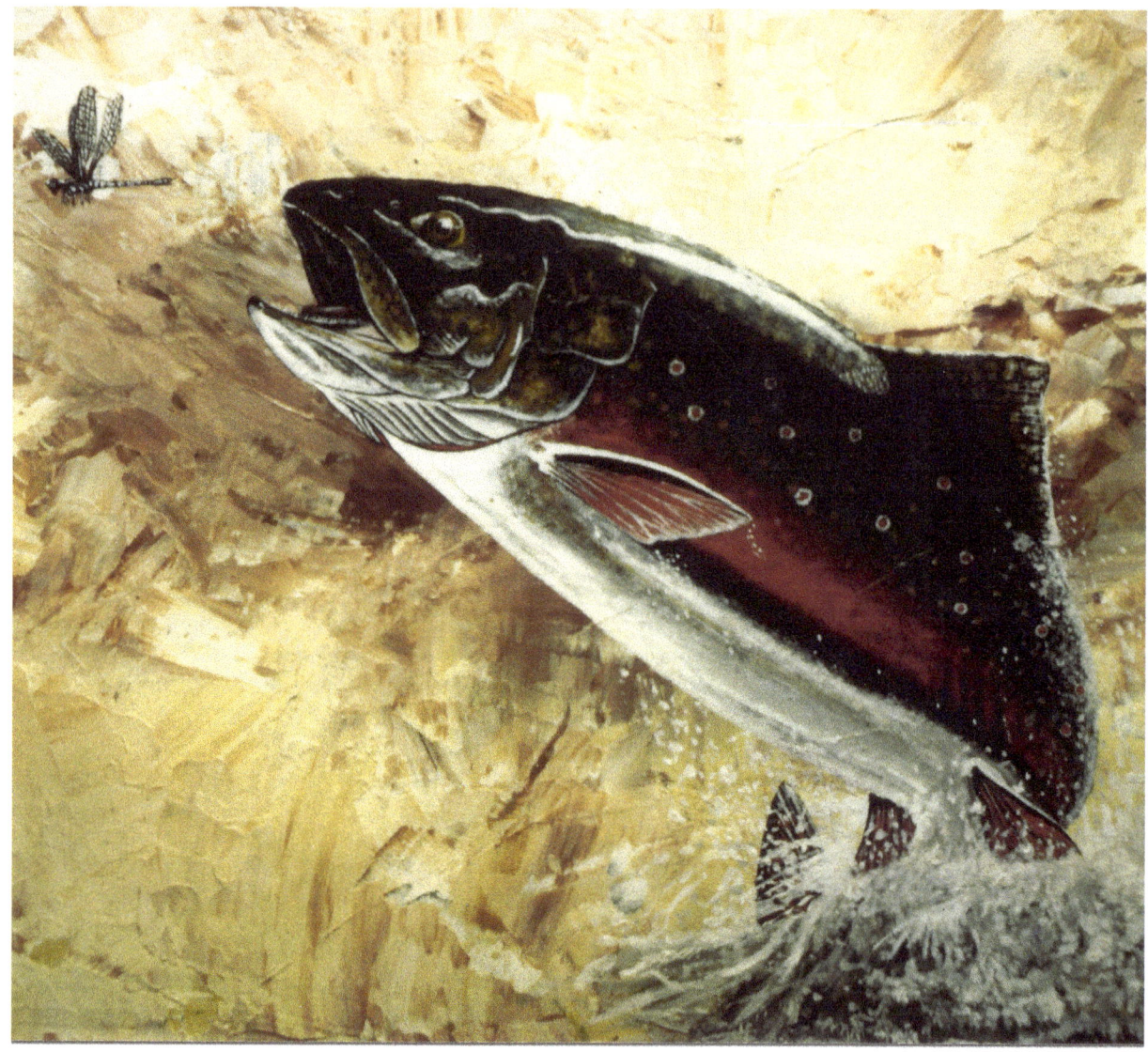

Brook Trout

I grew up in a place called Pleasant Valley, Winona, Minnesota, where we lived on a ten-acre parcel. Through the property was an ice-cold clear creek that ran through the middle. This was my home from the time I was twelve years old to when I was about nineteen. I learned to love trout fishing. It was perfect.

The main source to the creek was an artesian well where the Aldinger's, Marty and Mike lived and of course their parents. They were roughly the same ages as my brother and I. Their parents had struck the artesian well when they were digging the foundation of their new home. In the big hole, water was bubbling up at a rapid pace producing many gallons a minute, thus contributing greatly to increase the flow of the creek. Well, they made a trout pond and filled it with brown trout, brook trout and rainbow trout.

Like many pets, these trout got big and fat and had babies. Yee Haw! I have many pictures taken with the fish I caught from this creek. One of the first I caught was about a five-pound brook trout. I caught it with hay bale twine and a heavy staple for a hook. I climbed a log he was under, dropped the staple under his big hooked snout and yanked him out of the water and onto the sand, jumping on him to make sure he did not get away. His length surpassed my shoulder width at twelve years old. I was very proud to catch dinner that day and every day when I can bring a meal to my family.

Trout fishing and many other types of fishing has been my passion since childhood. Fresh crappie or blue gill made into crisp little taco filler that makes your mouth water. Yum! Sushi is also a favorite of mine, I make with tuna, yellowtail, salmon and other ocean species. This love has inspired many of my paintings, as you will see. This is a beautiful freshwater specimen of the trout family weighing in at an approximate max weight of twenty pounds. It loves cold, fast moving water, brooks and streams, which was just what I had running through my back yard as a kid.

My dad bought and built a three-bedroom home on this property in the early 70's. We made that place into a nice little horse property with a barn and corrals fenced off to keep the livestock in. It was a lot of work for a thirteen year old with a broken arm, but looking back it was all worth the hard work. Besides, the arm healed over time and all that work helped strengthen and straighten my arm. Living there about 6 years as a teenager, I had plenty of opportunity to fish in a pristine stream in South Eastern Minnesota, the land of ten thousand lakes and a million streams. Almost all of them teaming with brook trout, brown trout and rainbow. A Fishing paradise for sure.

My most memorable experience was when we were first building the house, I was around thirteen and my cousin Warren and I went for a walk along the stream. It was perfectly clear, you could see all the way to the bottom, there under a log I spot a big brook trout, the king of the creek. He was not afraid; he just sat there not trying to hide. He made it easy for me to see him. With his hooked nose hanging over his lower jaw, it was obvious he was a mature male. All excided with adrenalin a flow I ran to the construction trash pile to see what I could find to catch him. I did not have a pole so I had to improvise. I found some twine string used for bailing hay or tying other things together and a staple, the thick strong ones they use for holding the tops of big boxes together, I bent it to form an eye at one end and hook at the other. I tied the twine to the eye with a granny knot, at the time I did not know any other to catch this fish and off to the creek I ran.

That big boy was still there under the log so I snuck up from down stream knowing they all ways face upstream unless disturbed. On my belly I crawled out onto the log, peeping over the edge, I could still see him. I lowered my hook under his hooknose with a big fat night crawler on it, one that I had dug up from under a log by the creeks edge. Nothing, no reaction what so ever, so I jiggled it, bobbed it and swam it to no avail. He would not take the bait for nothing.

Frustrated I jerked the line up and it caught under his hooked snout. As his body came out of the water I flung him towards the bank and in midair, he came off the hook. He hit the bank with a slap, slappidy slap, I dove on top of him gabbing him by the gills and lifting him up, he was for sure a prize for me to take home for dinner. The biggest fish I ever caught at the time weighing in at approximately five pounds a trophy for a brook trout.

I felt proud. I took him up to the house to show off my catch to my parents and all the workers none of which ever caught a brook trout this big before. My family ate well that night. He was a plentiful amount of fresh fish, straight from mother earth, to satisfy the hunger from a hard days work. That was not the only big book trout I have caught in an unusual manner.

On another occasion a few years later, we had heavy rains one summer day and the creek rose into a small river, the water no longer clear, it was full of mud and debris. It's fast moving sludge clogged our culverts, which allowed water to flow under the dirt bridge that spanned the creek. Water was flowing over the top of the bridge approximately 8 inches deep at the deepest. I saw the back of a fish trying to swim up stream fighting the current. His back and dorsal fins were sticking out of the water, the strong current was winning as he was slowly forced backward. Instantly with out thinking of the dangers I ran out to the fish, swiped it up out of the water, and up on the bank like a bear might have swatted it out of the water. Again, I ran up and jumped on the fish a technique I still use today. This big Brook Trout was approximately thirteen pounds.

Sometimes they are just that big and you just have to jump on them so they do not get away. Where were these big trout coming from; well, Aldinger's pond of course. In heavy rains, the pond would over flow and fish would escape. These trout were being hand fed and were not too afraid of humans. The Brown Trout were of substantial size, up to 30 pounds. That pond was the source of all the fish in the creek. I have never caught one of those 30 pounders yet but it is on my list of things to do. I fished that creek from beginning to end over the years, all fifteen miles of it. I have caught literally hundreds of trout over time. For me this place was perfect, any real anglers' paradise. Water is everywhere; it is no wonder the state bird of Minnesota is the mosquito.

Rainbow Trout

Another beautiful addition to the species of trout is the Rainbow Trout. This one being the most abundant strain, it makes its home in lakes, rivers and streams. It also goes out to sea, when driven by instinct to do so. When it reaches the ocean, it will live out its life until maturity. Then as an adult, it will go back to the creek or river from which it was born and swim up stream to spawn as a Steelhead salmon. The Rainbow is the most commonly used trout for stocking lakes and rivers in North America.

I happen to live by the largest natural lake in Southern California. The Rainbows just started biting recently. The department of natural resources stocks it on a regular basis with Rainbow trout. All other species that live in the lake, with the exception of the mosquito fish, are natural to this lake. There are Bass, Blue Gill, Black Crappie and a form of Catfish called the Bull Head. On a rare occasion a Gold fish is caught, a by-product of public interference. I saw one swim by one day and it must have been at least six or seven pounds, which is big for a Gold fish, but that is the lake full of great natural resources.

I fish this place a lot, in most cases I drive by it twice a day to and from work. I cannot help myself sometimes I just have to stop now and again, sometimes three to five times a week, when the fish are biting to cast a line. This is another nice place to live surrounded by forest, lakes and streams, a virtual oasis for Southern California. Most of Southern California is desert or dry mountains.

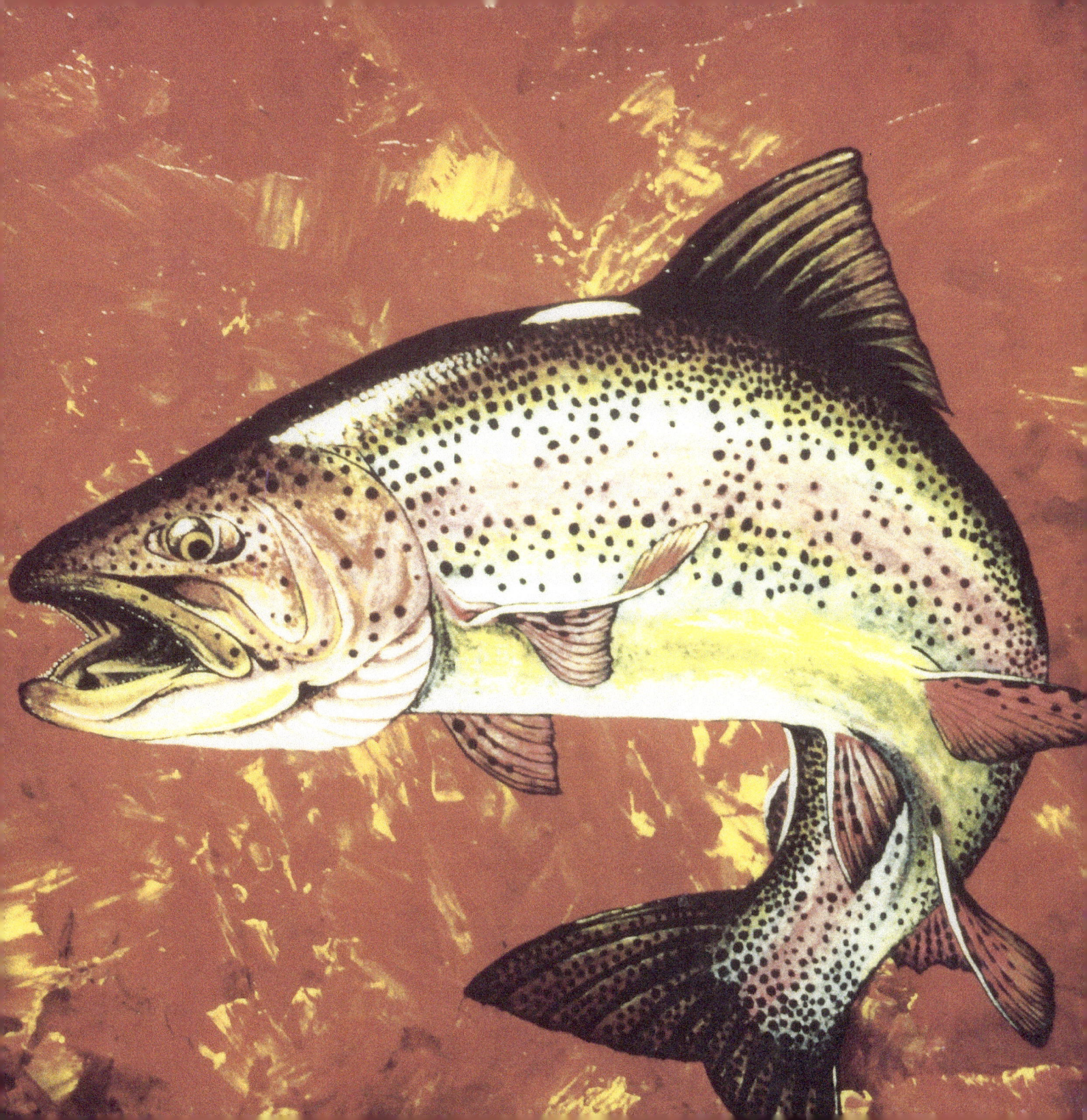

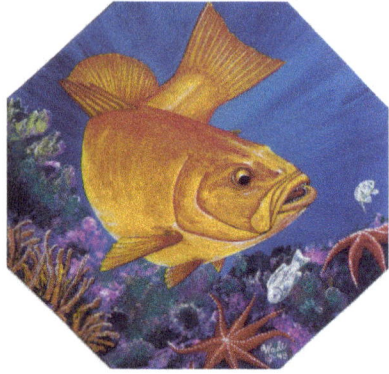

Golden Grouper

Leopard Grouper

On another fine trip to Bahia De Los Angeles, three friends and I took my boat to the north end of Smith Island an extinct volcano. At this end of the island was another small island known as bird rock that was covered with mounds of white bird droppings like icing on a muffin. Between the two islands was a channel where there was an under water cliff that we fished in hopes we would catch some Grouper. That day we did and they where hitting good on three-inch metal yoyo jigs, yellow and white in color, we were being nailed by four to six pound freight trains. Every now and then, a larger one would hit and take the jig slamming you against the rail. Needless to say, you usually lost that one. They would take it back to there hole in the under water cliff and just sit there, eventually the line would break from rubbing on the volcanic rock and bye bye jig.

Just one of the things you should be prepared for on a Baja trip, bring extra tackle you will need it. This day I got lucky and caught a Golden Grouper, which is a leopard grouper in an albino phase, this is a very rare catch. Several local anglers saw what I caught and called me the golden child in Spanish and told me this was a very good omen, and that I was blessed by mother earth to be given that gift. Just in case you have never ate fresh caught grouper it is the best pan-fried delight you could ask for after a long hot hard day of fishing. Fillet that beauty then dip the fillets in egg then in cracker crumbs drop them in the frying pan with a little butter then cook to a golden brown, season to taste and voila a meal fit for a king.

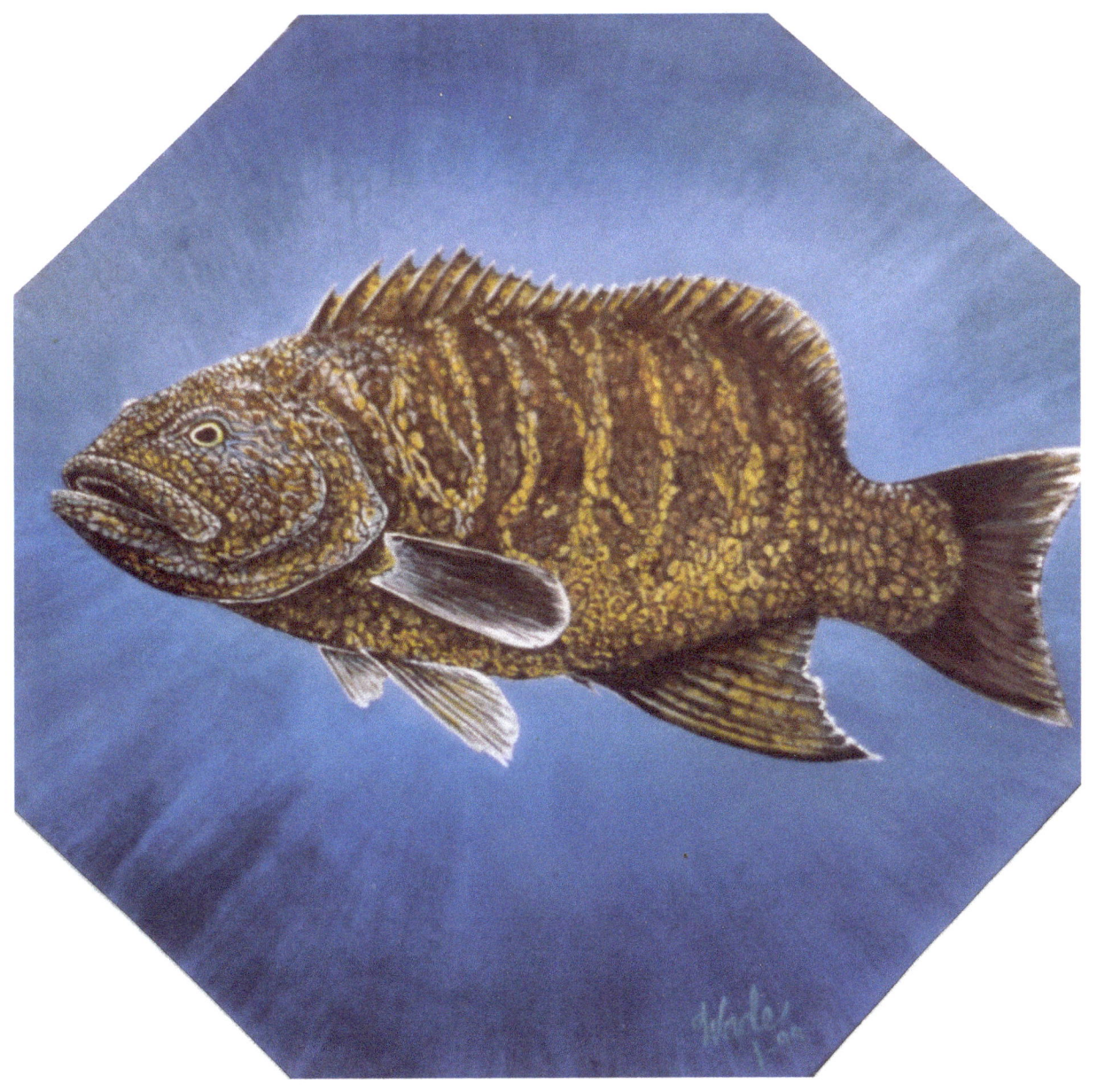

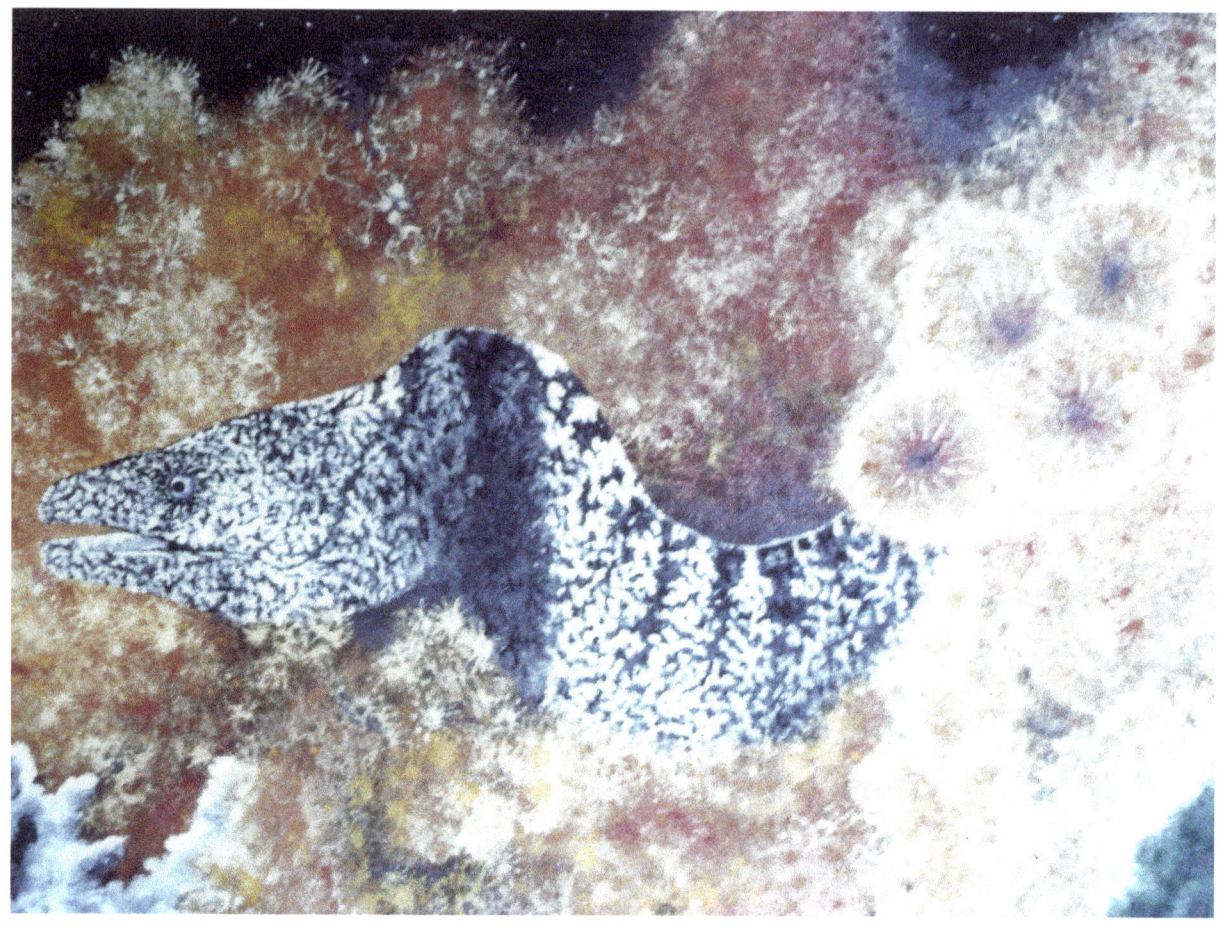

The Morey Eel

This painting is number one, but is not really the first of my paintings. There are a few previous paintings I have done that were not numbered. This is one of only a small number of oil paintings that I have done. The rest are acrylic or mixed oil background with acrylic foreground. Needless to say, most of my art is wild life, specifically animals of all types. Not much different from a cave man, some would say. Hunt, fish, gather and garden; I have not strayed far from Neanderthal. I live in a cinder block house with animals all over the place, from floor to ceiling. Kind of like a cave man. At least so says my wife.

The Morey Eel can reach lengths of six feet. I have never knowingly approached one while snorkeling, but with their excellent ability to hide amongst the coral one never knows. From a photo on a calendar featuring ocean fauna my inspiration came. It was such a great picture I was inspired to paint my own rendition of a Morey Eel. There are a few of my paintings that I have had no real life encounters, just a beautiful photograph.

There are still critters I have met that I have not painted yet, probably because it takes me so long to paint them. I am slow and meticulous when I paint. I must be happy and feeling creative to be able to sit long enough to do the work. I am usually quite active so having the time to do the work is slim, but I manage at times to do it. Now you think I have a hard time taking the time to paint. Imagine what it takes to get me to write!

No, I am not in jail. I contracted the first planned job ever as a general contractor, the biggest I have ever gotten. I am happy and most of the work, like 95% is done by sub-contractors. I am the babysitter of the job. I arrange, organize, and set things up for the next phase. I meet with people, write checks, call for inspections and deal with all the daily problems. So when I have downtime on the job, I write. I have thought about writing this book for about ten years, but never took the time to actually sit down and do it. Well, now is a good time.

I am just an average person who had an idea, which led to a goal, and then to another and slowly over time I achieved those goals. At this moment, I am rich, not with money, but love. I have succeeded in surrounding myself with positive, good people who care about my wife and I. They are great people. This is a good thing. Without this love, creativeness would be stifled. It is hard to be relaxed when you are angry, upset or stressed. If only all humankind could feel this peace and share it with each other, there would be no war, no murder, no rape, no greed, no stealing, etc. I guess that would be a perfect world and I do not see that happening. So I feel blessed that in this time, for me, I have found true happiness. Life is good.

The Guardian Angel

In this painting of four dolphins, which was done for my sister, the dolphins represent my sis, her husband and daughter and son. John was the youngest of her children, making the smallest dolphin him. He was just a baby at the time, maybe 4 years old. Her daughter Sarah (seventeen) is the one not quite full grown with Kathy my sis in the middle with her faithful husband, John, at their side. My sister was dying; she had pancreatic cancer, mortality rate is one hundred percent. She asked me in July to paint her some dolphins for her birthday in October. I did not finish it in time for her birthday. Still in November when I went to see her, I had not finished it. I am not quite sure, but everything happens for a reason. She died when I was there in Minnesota, almost as if she waited and put off death until she could say goodbye. I am crying now as I write this down, the memory of her still so vivid and sad. Goodbye dear sis, I love you. When I returned home to California, I set to finishing her painting. I could not stop crying while I diligently painted using my tears to moisten my brush. I painted the image of Kathy in the dolphin that represented her. I want her remembered as everyone's guardian angel and for being the wonderful daughter, the great mother and the loving sister that she was.

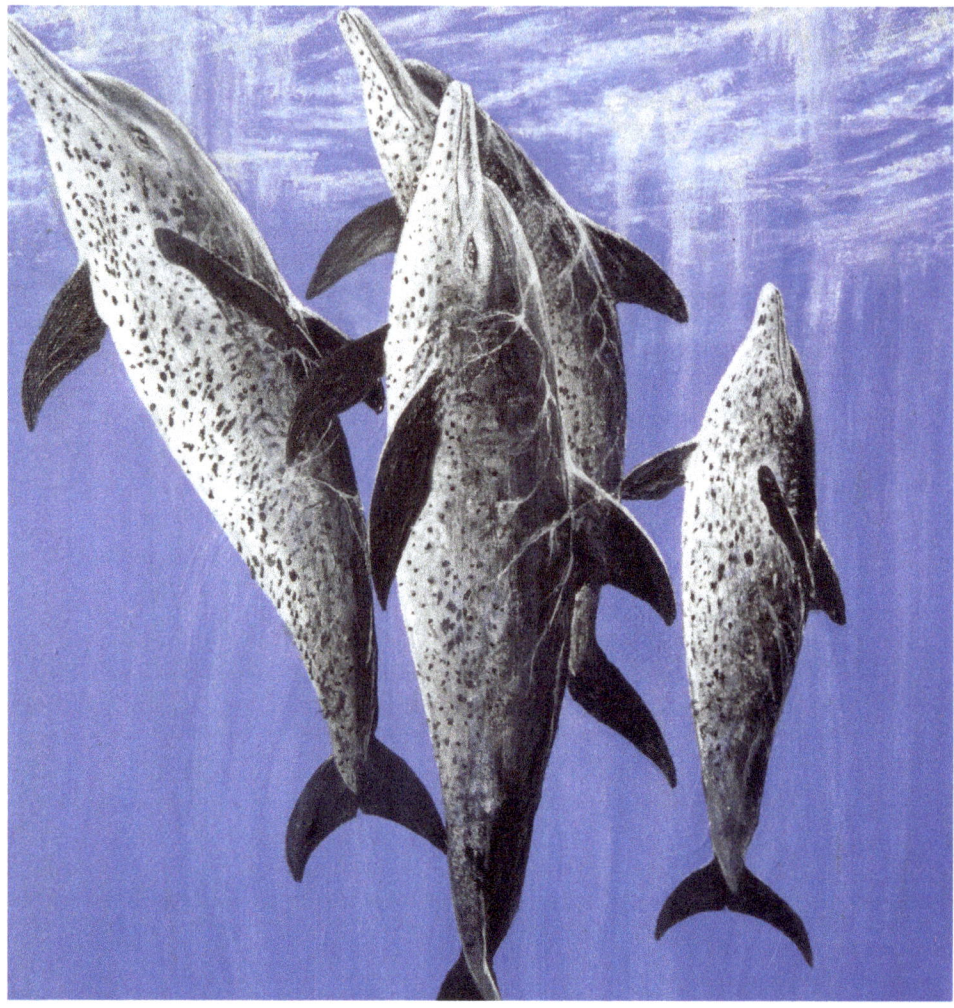

So many things have happened to me in my life. I should not be alive or at least messed up good but alas, my guardian angel watched out for me today she protected me from harm. I was digging a trench for the plumber and I jumped on the shovel with both feet. The shovel kicked out and away I went, falling backwards over form boards and into a footing with only a few scrapes and bruises. I came out of this mishap well and no worse for the wear and tear.

Another time, long ago, when I was seventeen, I was lying on the back of my sister's appaloosa stud while she was preparing for a ride. I was facing the sky with my head towards the head of the horse. My sister and I were talking when all of a sudden "the horse" took off towards the barbed wire fence, which enclosed his domain. The fence was made of four barbed, barbed wire and eight inches apart with six wires, a formidable combo. I spun around on his back grabbing on with my legs and holding this small crop of hair left at the base of his crew cut mane. Away he went towards the fence at full gallop. Me, anticipating him to jump the fence, I held on to no avail. Instead of jumping off which would of been the smart thing to do, I held on. As he hung a sharp left towards the gate, I continued going straight forward. I flew right into the sturdy parallel strands of barbed wire. I put my hands forward like a diver and aimed at an opening in the fence and closed my eyes anticipating certain injury. I went through that eight-inch gap of wire without a scratch. My cowboy boot was hanging by the toe on a barb four strands up. I looked up to the sky and thanked the woman who helped me come into this world. Not my mother, but a little old woman, a midwife in a small town in Minnesota who died from a stroke one day after helping deliver me. However, that is a whole other story. Thank you, my guardian angel!

I have had several experiences that have lead me to believe that in deed I do have my very own guardian angel. I had fished the channel between Catalina and Los Angeles many times, however on this particular trip an acquaintance from Minnesota John, with whom I grew up with worked for the same company as my mother, only the office he worked at was here in Los Angeles, that's how I knew he was out here "small world really".

I picked him up at his house before the crack of dawn, we wanted to hit the docks early, and we were ready for the adventure ahead. We made it to what we called "the fishing zone" which we both determined by the boil we spotted. It was a feeding frenzy, a whole bunch of bigger fish pushing a big school of small bait fish to the surface. Of course, this brought the birds in too. Hundreds of Sea Gulls diving in to the water and swimming up to the surface with their beaks full, some others were sitting on the top of the water just reaching out and grabbing the little swimmer bys. Their breakfast was much appreciated, easy pickings brought to them from the bigger fish below. We quickly baited up and the bite was on, the fish responsible for that boil were three to four pound Mackerel. We were using light weight line so hooking these little fighters was fun, what a hoot.

As we were fishing, the skies were darkening. All around us and where we were, the sun was still shining. Thunder and lighting began to take over Los Angeles and surrounding us on all sides. The sky tuned black as we watched the storm growing in power. As we continued to fish, we saw seven waterspouts towards Catalina Island. Three at one time all of which when they hit the ocean they took up water, they turned from grey to white and then dissipated. That was an incredible sight.

Where we were fishing the sun continued to shine, it was great. We thought about packing it up and heading home because of the storm but we thought we would stay and stick it out as long as we could. The weather remained fine where we were not a drop of rain fell on us. All the while nature's wrath raised havoc through out Los Angeles and the surrounding areas. It was like being in the eye of a hurricane. We did not see a drop of rain until we got home. It was as if the heavens were looking out for us, perhaps my Guardian Angel.

There are literally dozens of experiences I could tell you about, concerning the times that I have come hazardously close to meeting my demise. For example, I have been shot with a twelve gage shot gun with out to much harm. I have had guns put to my head several times. I have had people try to stab me with knives and one person tried to stab me with a pitch fork another person tried to spear me with a home made spear. I had a chainsaw shoved between my legs catching me at the inseam, it cut out a swath of denim from my crotch to my belt loop, to my relief not a scratch and I still have my junk. The list could go on but that is for another book.

Now you know why I tend to believe I have my own guardian angel. I also believe my guardian angel has sent me my own angel here on earth that being my wife Jo.

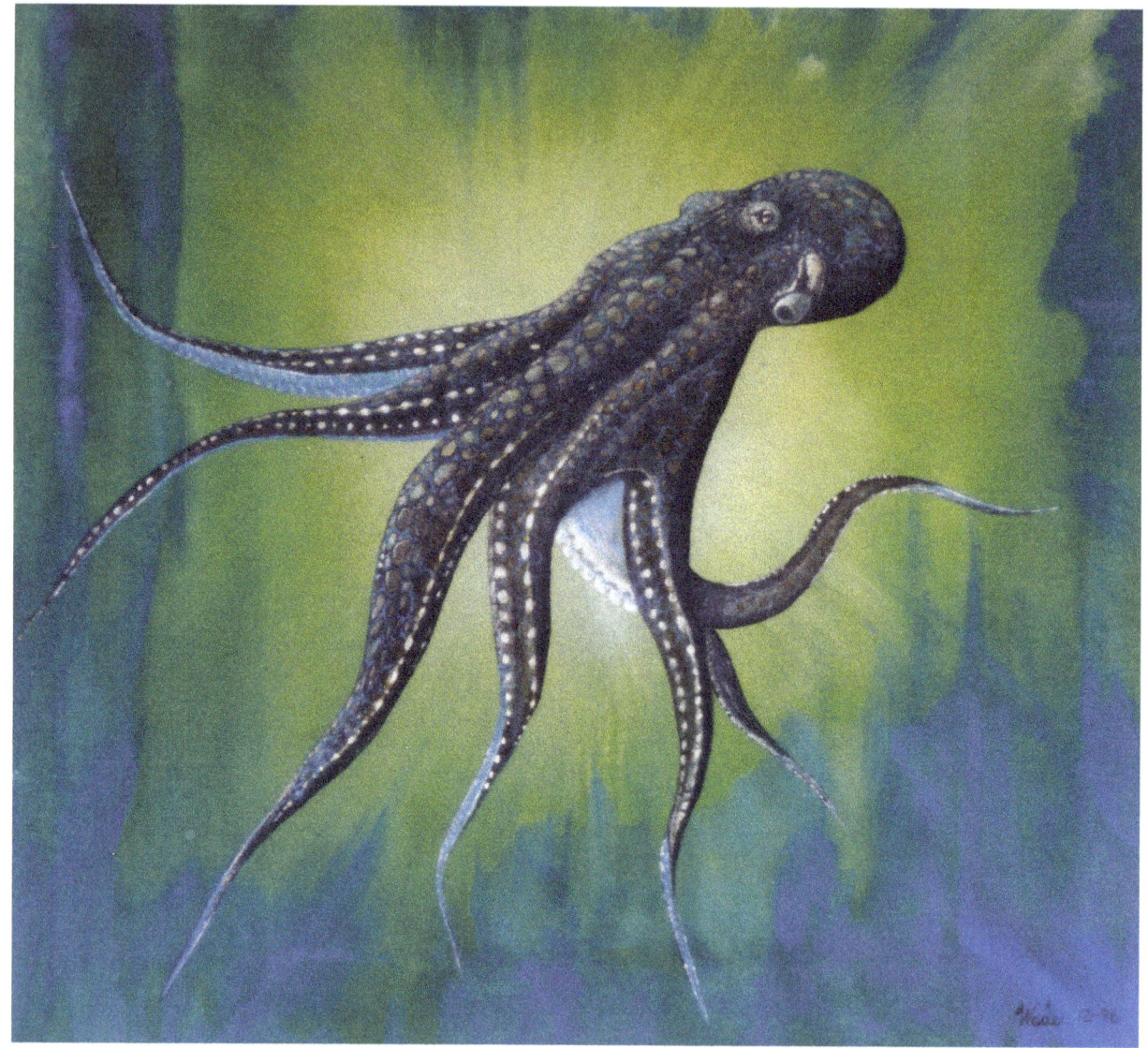

The Blue Ringed Octopus

This Cephalopod is small and beautiful however, this little guy packs a deadly punch. Their small size of five to seven inches and weighing in at a whole .92oz a full-grown specimen could easily fit in my wives hand. This little critters poison (tetrodotoxin) is so strong that with a single bite, which administers approximately, one milligram of toxin can paralyze and kill an adult person in minutes. They also have a second toxin they use to hunt crab, fish and mollusks; this toxin is harmless to humans. When this small octopus is calm or at rest it is grey or beige with light brown patches. However, when they feel threatened or agitated its fifty to sixty blue rings pulsate and glow while its body becomes bright yellow. This makes them one of the most sought after octopi for photographers. They are not only pursued for their beauty they are also hunted for their powerful muscular-neurotoxins. There are twelve different species named by the amount of rings they have. This large headed two-eyed cephalopod has two rows of suction cups on its eight arms, which makes it a formidable predator for its size. Therefore, if you ever get to see one remember you can look but do not touch.

The Humboldt Squid

Unfortunately, as of this time in my life I have not yet painted a picture of one of the most formidable predators of the sea, the Humboldt Squid. However, I would like to share this experience with you.

The sun rose on the Sea of Cortez in a bright orange red glow, beams of light came through the distant clouds in an array of colors from yellow to deep blood red making a spectacular sunrise. It was calm on the sea; the water was like glass, perfect for fishing. The guide, Jose, was tying on a jig for the bass on the bottom, which was about three hundred feet down where he stopped the sixteen-foot panga. The drift would bring us across an underwater ridge that came up from the depths to zero feet at low tide and the rocky top would expose itself to the air and unsuspecting boaters. Many of who did smash into the rocks as the tide rushed out and their boats came in contact with the jagged pinnacles. The place was Punta Rojo, thus named probably because of all the blood that has been spilled in the water there.

I was set up with a rock cod rig, five hooks, eighty pound test line and a two pound weight on the end to get down to the bottom fast with out the currant drifting your line out so you never hit bottom. The bait was pieces of sand bass caught the night before while the boat was moored in the bay. On the first drop I was nailed, bam, bam, bam! It was a multitude of fish attacking my baited hooks. I immediately set the hooks and began reeling in what seemed like a hundred pounds of wriggling mass. As the fish were thrashing to get off the hooks in every different direction, I was pulling up with the rod to bring up the fish and reeling as I brought the rod tip down. Coming up from the depth of three hundred feet this was a lot of work. You only gain about three feet of line each time you pull and reel. About a hundred fifty feet up from the bottom, the weight tripled as something big attached itself to the end of my line, pulling the rod and I to the edge of the boat. I looked over at the other anglers and they were all in the same predicament. Everyone except

Jose had the look of surprise and pain on their face. Jose was laughing as he yelled out "Diablo rojo"! This means Red Devil in Spanish.

Jose was the first to bring one of these red devils to the boat. It was about five feet long, maybe fifty to sixty pounds and rapidly changing color from red to white and then back to red. As I stared in awe at the biggest squid I have ever seen, it squirted me in the face with a jet of water and ink in an effort to get away. What I saw was a snake like projectile of water jump out and hit me in the face. I was covered in black slime that would not wash off and everyone was laughing. With my hand, I tried to wash it off but it was not working, so I grabbed a rag to remove the black goo from my face. The front of my clothes were black, a stain that does not come out, it is permanent. Jose, one hand holding the rod, the other a short two-foot gaff pulled the sea monster on board. He quickly pulled out his knife, cut off the tentacled head and threw it back in the ocean, explaining to us that it contained a beak like a parrot and could take a bite out of you the size of a golf ball.

Meanwhile I continued to gain on the Volkswagen I was reeling in and finally got it to the boat. Another Humboldt Squid and a couple of rockfish with heads still attached to the other hooks. With a little help from Jose, I landed the squid in the panga with its head facing me. Instantly it shot out two long tentacles that grabbed my leg. Its body slid across the deck as it was coming to take a bite out of me. Instinctively I slammed my rod butt between the tentacles and my leg to avoid being bitten. Jose reached out and cut off the two tentacles with his knife and quickly moved to the beheading on the next cut. Laughing as he said, "Good reaction, you just saved yourself a lot of pain". Then he grabbed the squids head and cut out the black beak to show us the razor sharp weapon. All the while, I still had these tentacles still stuck to my leg. As I pulled them off, they left cartilage like circular hooked rings stuck in my leg. I picked them out and looked at them amazed at the fact that they came out of the suckers. They left bloody rings on my leg where they were attached.

Jose and I were the only two to land our squid. Usually they grab your fish, eat their fill and let go without being hooked. Jose sliced the squid body in half removing the innards, leaving a slab of meat about one inch thick, four feet long and four feet wide. Then he sliced us off a couple of small pieces, part of the squid that almost bit me, he popped a piece in his mouth and handed me the other. I reluctantly put it in my mouth and began to chew and chew. It was very tough and tasted like an unusual fishy cream flavor, leaving a slimy sensation coating the inside of my mouth. I almost threw up as I spat it out into the water. I hope that it tasted better cooked because raw was nasty.

Do to the practice of shark finning and the depletion of the world's shark populations the Humboldt squid is rapidly becoming the dominant predator of the sea, prompting more encounters with humans.

Sea Lions

In July 1989, I was hired by Mira Costa College in San Diego to take my boat to Bahia De Los Angeles on an eighteen-day biology trip. This was a memorable trip, all expenses paid by the college, not that the others trips were not memorable. My job was to escort students and teachers out to the islands, for a period of time, to do their field study on whatever island they were on.

There are a lot of islands in this area because at one time there had been a lot of volcanic activity. Because of this violent past, there are a lot of under water caves, out crops and pinnacles for sea life to flourish. All around you,

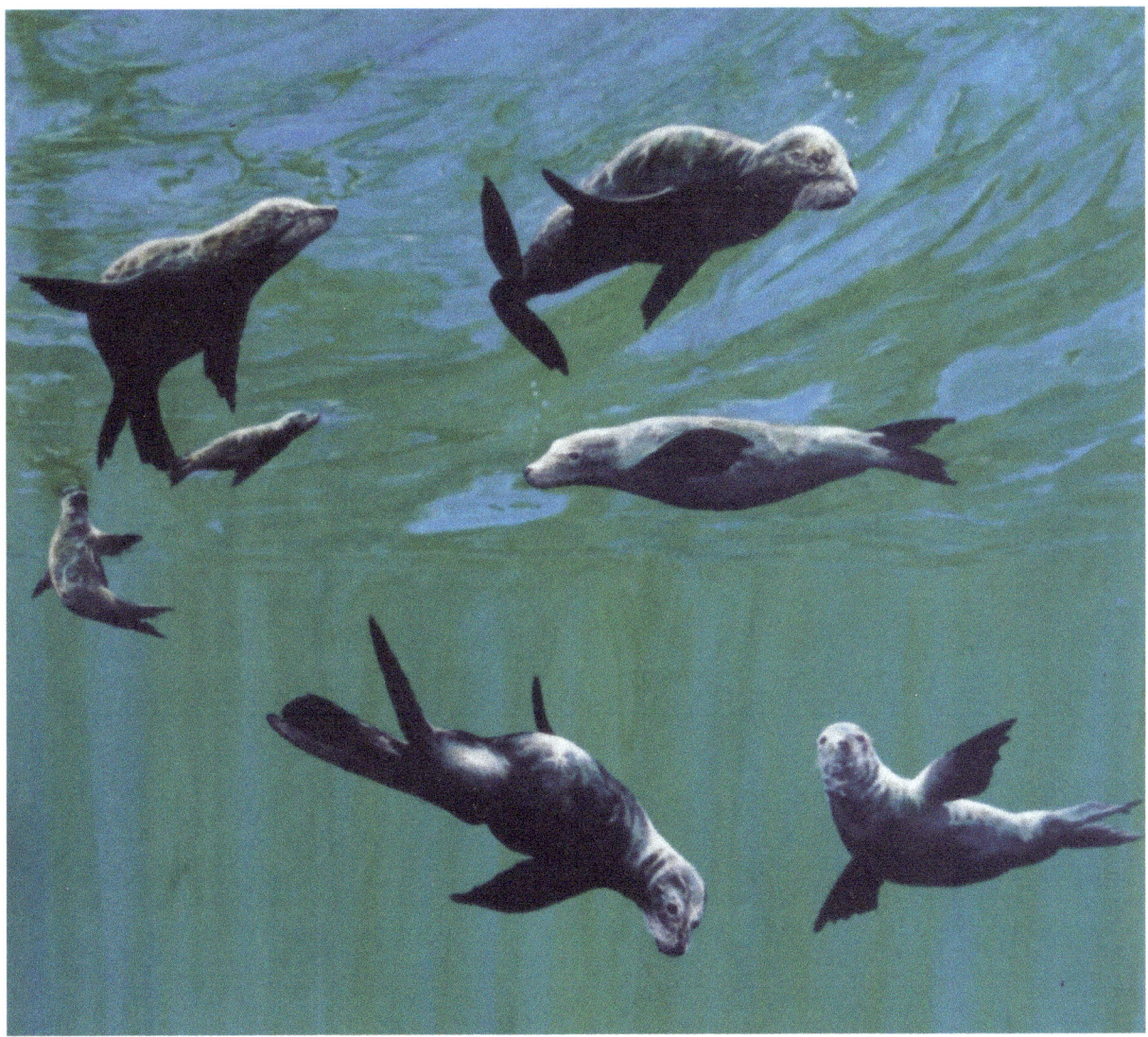

the area teems with life. I have been fishing in the Atlantic Ocean, the Pacific Ocean and many places in between, but nothing compares to the Sea of Cortez.

I have seen sea lions, dolphin and birds of every coastal species in this fantastic oasis. The pelicans there will come right aboard to steal the fish you just caught. Huge grouper, sea bass, tuna yellowtail, Humboldt squid, grey whales, and turtles; the list goes on and on.

Many of my experiences at this heaven of mine inspired paintings, like the sea lions. On this particular trip I got close to many of the seas awesome inhabitants.

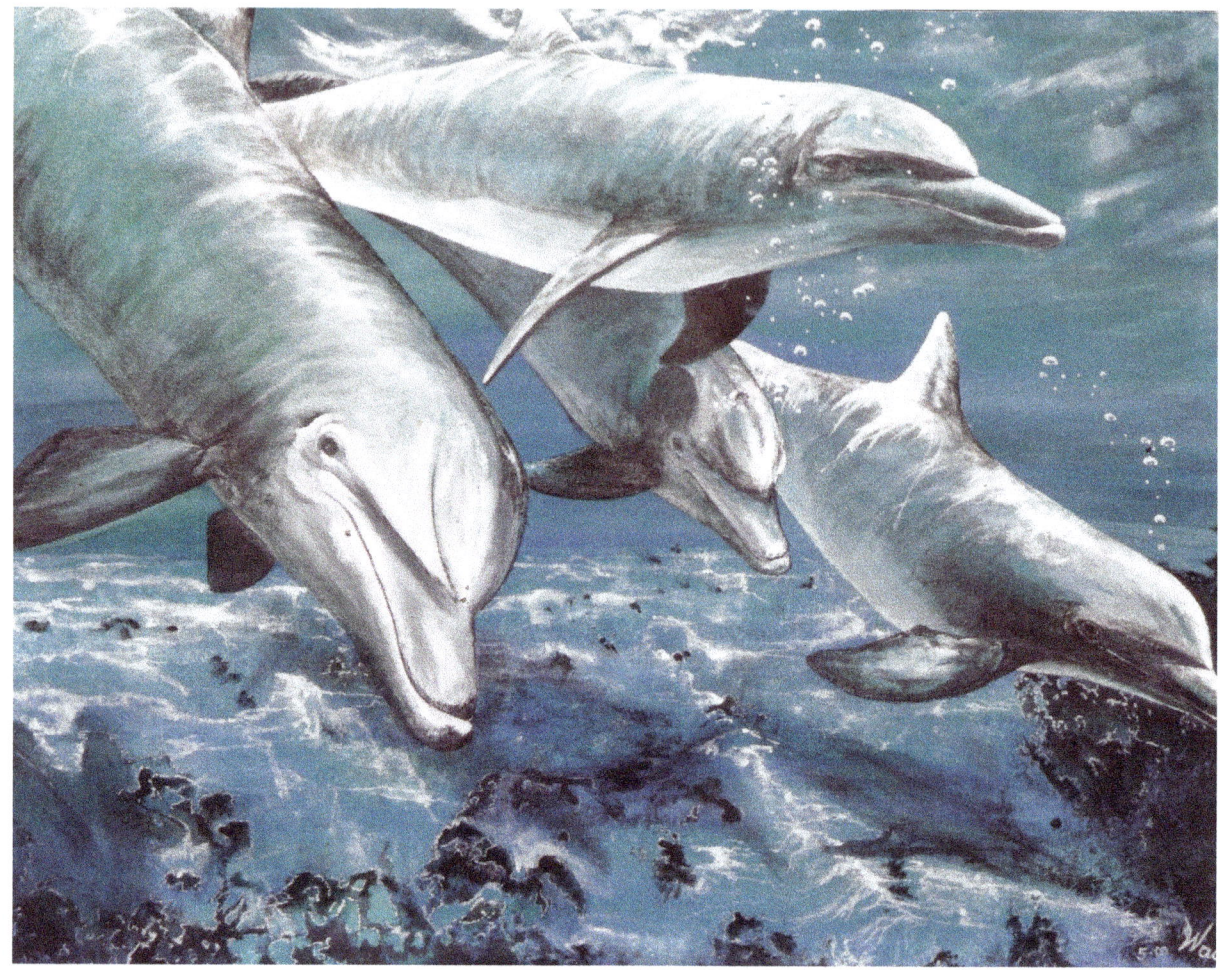

The common Dolphin

On one sunny day, uh, what am I thinking, they were all sunny and one hundred plus degrees. It was cooler when you got farther out to the sea. You could feel the wall of heat end and the wall of cool relief begin as you entered the cooler climate of the open ocean. At the end of a long day, just the opposite would take place as you approached the land. That desert heat loomed over the land as if a giant oven was turned on.

This day out to one of the islands, I went with a boatload of students. Along the way, we came across a pod of dolphins that was literally numbered in the hundreds. There were so many, without exaggeration acres of them. My crew and I were right in the midst of this gigantic pod. It was great watching the dolphins watching us, they swam right next to the boat full of curiosity, and it was obvious they were checking us out. I slowed the boat down to a stop so everyone could get in the water with the dolphins except for me I had to stay behind to operate the boat. Everyone in the water was able to touch one or more as they swam close enough to touch. It was amazing to see such a spectacle, one of many to come. We finally made it out to the sea lion island where many a sea lion lived and hunted, including great white sharks.

Again, I brought the boat to a halt about a hundred yards from the island shore. Sea lions covered the island. They were everywhere, in the water and on land, it smelled of dead fish. We could hear their calls to one another, it sounded like barking. They played out there ocean existence in front of us. There was a big bull on alert. He kept an eye on us as we entered their domain, you could tell he was looking over his family with concern ready to protect then if the need called for it. It seemed as though he was thinking," Who are these strange beings invading our home". "I should beware" and goes into a defensive mode. He entered the water with a huge splash, all six hundred pounds of fat and testosterone ready for battle.

By now, there are all but a few people in the water with them, adorned with goggles, snorkels and flippers. They gawked through their glass covers as the sea lions curiously swam around them, too afraid to get too close. They made sure to keep a distance of ten to fifteen feet. I dropped anchor, pulled out my favorite jig and proceeded to fish, cranking a jig for grouper or sheep head. Sometimes you would catch a triggerfish or two using this method and an array of other species depending on the structure of the bottom. This was rocky, a perfect hangout for the groupers. I caught a few small ones, three to four pounds while the swimmers took their chances with the big bull sea lion. Luckily, there were no injuries or deaths that day. All of us got to get the up close and personal with these dog like ocean mammals. Yet just one more awesome day at the Sea of Cortez, ending with a fresh fish dinner caught by yours truly.

Soon after that incredible day, I had another encounter with an amazing creature, the grey whale. On another excursion out to the extinct volcano, they call Smith Island. I dropped the students off on the south end of the island to hike there way to the top. This could take up a good part of the day. Leaving me time to head to the north end of the island. I knew this to be a great spot for fishing,

The grouper was my main target. Many times before I had fished this spot. At the north end is a small island called Bird Rock; this rock is where many aquatic birds rest and make their home. The majority of the rock is enshrouded with bird droppings. You can imagine the smell. The fishing is well worth the temporary stench, luckily, after awhile you become immune to it. There is a cliff off one side of this island combo under water and a myriad of big grouper make there home amongst the holes, pockets and caves that adorned this under water paradise. I was out to get at least one or two for dinner; well that was what I hoped for anyway. However, a forty-foot grey whale decided to try to make a new friend and would not leave me alone.

There were many in the area around this end of the island. A mother and calf were breaching less than a hundred yards from me and a single whale farther out was doing the same as mama and calf. It became commonplace for me to see this act many times over the hours. I was there by myself with the exception of one curious grey whale, male or female, I couldn't tell, I very much enjoyed seeing this giant, from time to time as close as four feet away. The whale's eye was the size of a small tea plate. We made eye contact many times, as it repeatedly went under my boat. It got to the point where I was poking him with my fishing pole and telling him to get lost. Saying "Hey I'm trying to fish here"! No harm was done to the leviathan. He probably never even felt it, because he did not respond at all. I felt no fear from this creature as it swam back and forth under the boat and coming up to the side to make eye contact, I truly felt like it was trying to be my new friend, I called him Buddy.

Though our friendship was short lived, the memory will last forever. I told Buddy that it was nice to meet you and have a long and fruitful life. It was time to go; I had to pick up the students. Well, I never forgot Buddy and I hope he never forgets me, even though I poked him with my fishing pole.

I have seen many whales like humpbacks in Mazatlan, Mexico; a mother and calf, a blue whale up close, maybe thirty yards. That is definitely close enough to get to the largest animal that ever lived; at one hundred forty five tons, these phenomenal beasts can reach lengths up to eighty-five feet long.

People pay to go out on boats just to see whales. I am lucky to have had friends with boats and then eventually get one of my own. This gave me the opportunity to see them and go fishing at sea without too much cost when I had little money and not much has changed. I always seem to have just enough to pay the bills; my phone always rings when I need it to and I end up getting some kind of work to pay for what I need. Everything seems to fall into place when I need it to. I have had a good life. Lucky some would say (namely me).

I do not have excess money or luxuries, but I do not need them. However, a new boat would be nice. All around me are the fruits of nature; from the land to the sea, I harvest the gifts that sustain my survival.

We live in the Garden of Eden. All you could want or need is all around us. All we have to do is make the effort to get it and you will reap the rewards of your efforts--well most of the time. If at first you do not succeed; try, try again. Do not give up! I have spent many years thinking about writing this book and now I am doing it. I am hoping that people will like my paintings and stories enough to buy it. Then maybe I will get what I need so I can pay the bills when I get older and have a place to rest in peace when I die.

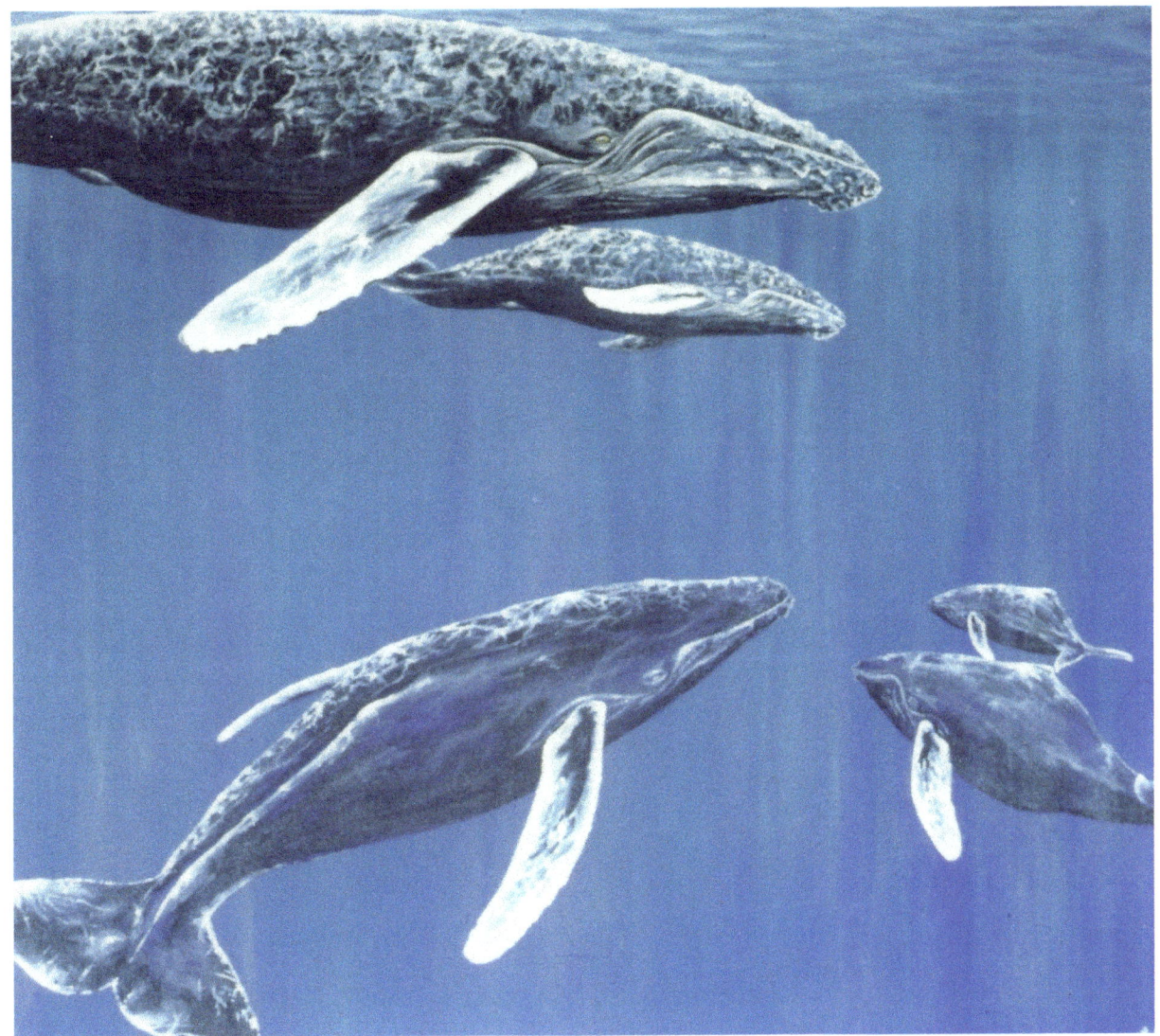

Humpback Whales

This is a painting of a pod of Humpback Whales.

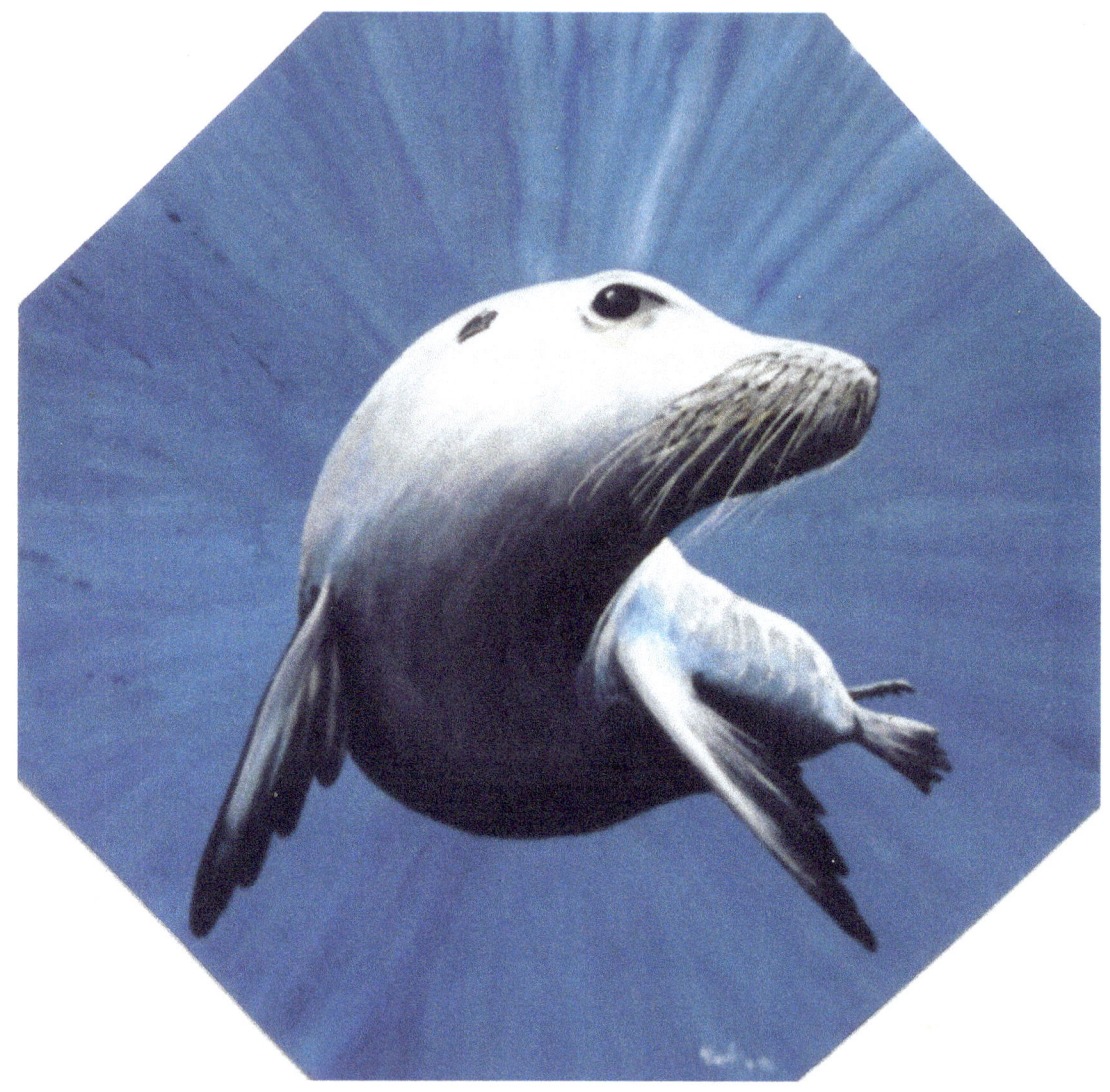

Sea Lion Octagon

Several paintings I have done are the shape of an octagon, as usual there is a story that goes with this anomaly in geometric shape compared to the others. I worked for MB construction in Van Nuys for approximately seventeen years. From the very start of my employment with this entity, we will refer to as Mike; the introductions to the stars began.

Mike got the job of contractor for many famous people. I met a lot of them over the years and worked around there homes. Arnold and Maria Schwarzenegger were the best customers for Mike. I was sent to their home a lot for handy work "Mr. Fixit". Their oldest daughter referred to me as The Handyman.

I did things on a regular basis for the Schwarzenegger's, sometimes doing tasks that took weeks at a time. At the time of this optical aberration in painting shapes, I was asked to build a custom doghouse for Strudel and Conan their two Golden Retrievers. They wanted the doghouse equipped with octagon shaped sliding Plexiglas windows. The size was, determined by me making samples for them to choose from. After they chose the size of window they wanted, the ones that were not used I threw canvas over and used them to paint on. One I used to paint the Sea Loin that you see in this book. I personally like this one a lot.

There was one time in particular when displaying my paintings I had for sale that was quite memorable. Luckily, a couple of restaurants allowed me to hang them in an effort to sell them. This Sea Lion painting made the channel seven news when they did a story on the actress that owned a restaurant in North Hollywood, which had five paintings of mine displayed on the walls. They featured this one on the news, "Woo Hoo"!!. It sold the next day, which was pretty cool; however, this did not turn into a trend. Sometimes things just come together perfectly; this was one of those times.

I know I am making a big deal over little things that have happened to me in my life, however life is full of little accomplishments and I appreciate them all. I am telling them to you as a way of telling you to appreciate all that is good, from the smallest details in life to your most sought after goal, from your dandelions in your yard to the air, water and soil etc. In doing so you will create a more positive way of thinking which leads to a happier and healthier life.

We will all meet our inevitable fate of death, so while we live we should try at least to enjoy it as much as possible out of what we are given. Every moment is a gift that is why we call it the present.

The Mountain Lions

Catamount is the name of this painting, it means cat of the mountains in old English. Other names for mountain lion are puma, cougar, painter and panther. This cat can reach lengths up to eight feet from head to tail and weigh up to two hundred pounds. It is usually nocturnal and solitary, seldom seen in the day.

It is a predator that hunts deer and other mammals by ambushing its prey from trees or rocky advantage points usually with a single bite to the neck. However, during their mating ritual, there is also biting of the neck, but these are just love bites, their way of having fore play. Mating may occur at any time through out the year however, most births happen in the warm summer months. The young cats remain with their mother approximately two years before they head out on their own. I have seen this cat four different times in the wild, three times during the day and once at night.

The most memorable of these sightings was the time I had a face-to-face encounter with one, we were less than four feet apart of one another. At the time, I was living on the edge of the Angeles National Forest in Southern California, in a place called Pine Canyon. My home was a small rustic one-bedroom cabin typical of the area.

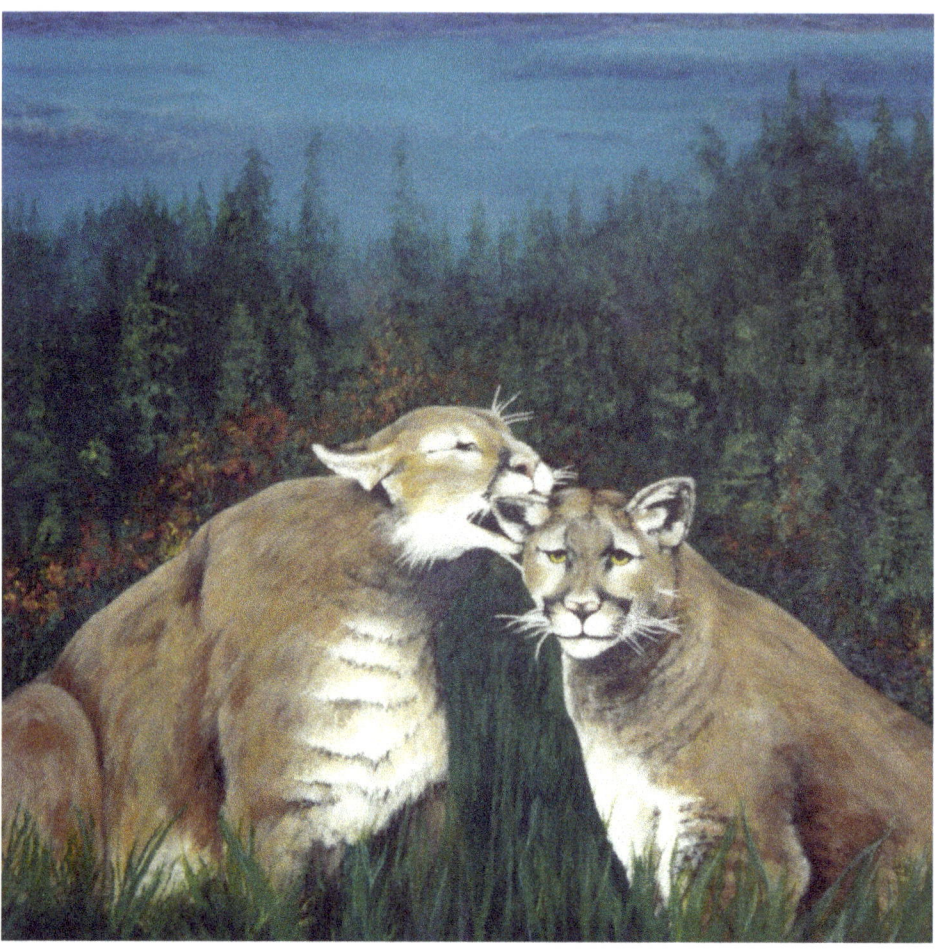

One evening just before sunset, my dogs alerted me by barking alarmingly at something. I knew it was not the typical bark of "Hey you have company" it was more like "WADE GET OUT HERE NOW". In somewhat of a rush I went out to see what all the fuss was about and saw the dogs at the four-foot fence on the east side of the yard.

I approached the fence and looked around to see why they were barking. Observing nothing, I then looked down at my dog Burbank who was looking straight out at the Blue Elder bush in front of me and to my surprise there it was, a mountain lion. Less than four feet away it was sitting there glaring me dead in the eyes. As I looked into its golden eyes in amazement, I saw no fear from this great cat only curiosity and the prospect of an easy meal. Frozen in my tracks I stood there staring into its eyes wondering what my next move was going to be as my heart was pounding wildly. Never braking eye contact I backed up approximately fifty feet from the cat because I knew their ability to leap was about thirty feet and my four-foot fence surely was not going to offer me any security.

At that point, I turned and ran into the house to get my twelve gage shot gun, which was loaded with OO buckshot and a flashlight because the light was fading fast. When I got back outside to protect my dogs and run that big critter out of there, it had already retreated across the road and into the wash. It was out of sight until I flashed the light over there and seen its glowing eyes staring back at me. I thought that maybe it had made its getaway instinctively knowing that three dogs and a human were bad odds or that maybe it had already experienced human contact and knew that it was in danger.

I feel lucky to have come that close to such a deadly predator without harm coming to any of us, me the cat or my dogs. I have seen them in the wild before, but never so up close and personal. I have a deep respect for this awesome predator and its ability to hunt me down and partake of my flesh. This brief encounter inspired me to paint one of nature's most agile carnivores.

Approximately a year and a half later Burbank and Red my two dogs, which are father and son, decided to break out of the yard and go for one of their nature outings without me. Burbank is Red's daddy; he is a mutt through and through, tawny in color and about fifty pounds. A brave little dog and one smart cookie, his curiosity sometimes gets him into trouble and he taught his son every thing he knows. Red is about a one hundred pounds and looks like a big red lab/ hound mix, but a mutt all the same. He is not as intelligent as his dad or as brave, but follows dad wherever he leads him. Which if he was smarter he would know it is not always a good idea to be lead around by his fearless daddy.

They took these nature adventures all too often without my permission or my guidance. On this particular day when they were not home by dark I opened the gate to allow easy access back in to the yard. Not one half hour later Red came running into the yard and straight into his doghouse, I thought that this was strange and decided to check on him. I crawled into the large doghouse to see if Red was hurt only to find him without injury but shaking like a leaf. Something definitely scared him and he would not leave the safety of his doghouse.

Shortly after, Burbank came running into the house and right up onto the couch he went. I remember saying to him "There you are you little mutt" and went outside to close the gate so that nothing else could come into the yard. Only then, did Red leave the safety of his doghouse and come into my house. When I went back in the house, I noticed Burbank wining in a high-pitched tone, which is his way of telling me something is wrong. I walked over to the couch where he was and immediately noticed him favoring his left rear leg. The leg was fillet wide open from his knee to his paw with the skin hanging off the back. The wound was so fresh it had not even had time to start bleeding. I rushed to get a towel to wrap his leg, as I was tending to his wound; it became clear to me that this was a slash caused by a mountain lion swiping his leg to take him down. He had dried blood on his back yet his wound was not bleeding. There was also fatty tissue on his back and I could smell deer on him.

My deduction was that he and Red had found a cougar kill and decided to have a snack and a roll. Well it was clear to me that the cougar did not want to share its feast with a couple of crafty K-9s. Therefore, Burbank must have been on the run from this cat and just barely made it into the yard. It was then I realized that when I closed the gate the cat must have been right there and I did not even know it. A shiver ran up my spine knowing that I could have been its next victim. Luckily, for Burbank there was no muscle or tendon damage, unluckily for me it cost me sixteen hundred dollars to fix his leg.

I believe this was the same cougar I met face to face a year and a half ago at the fence because they are known to make rounds in their territory on a regular basis and do not tolerate other mountain lions in their territory.

I saw this lion one more time a few months later. My dogs were acting up again and I went out to check with my flashlight and shot gun in hand. As I searched the darkness at the back of the property, I spotted it walking slowly up a fire road towards the water tank. I bid it adieu and brought my dogs in the house for the night never to see that cat again.

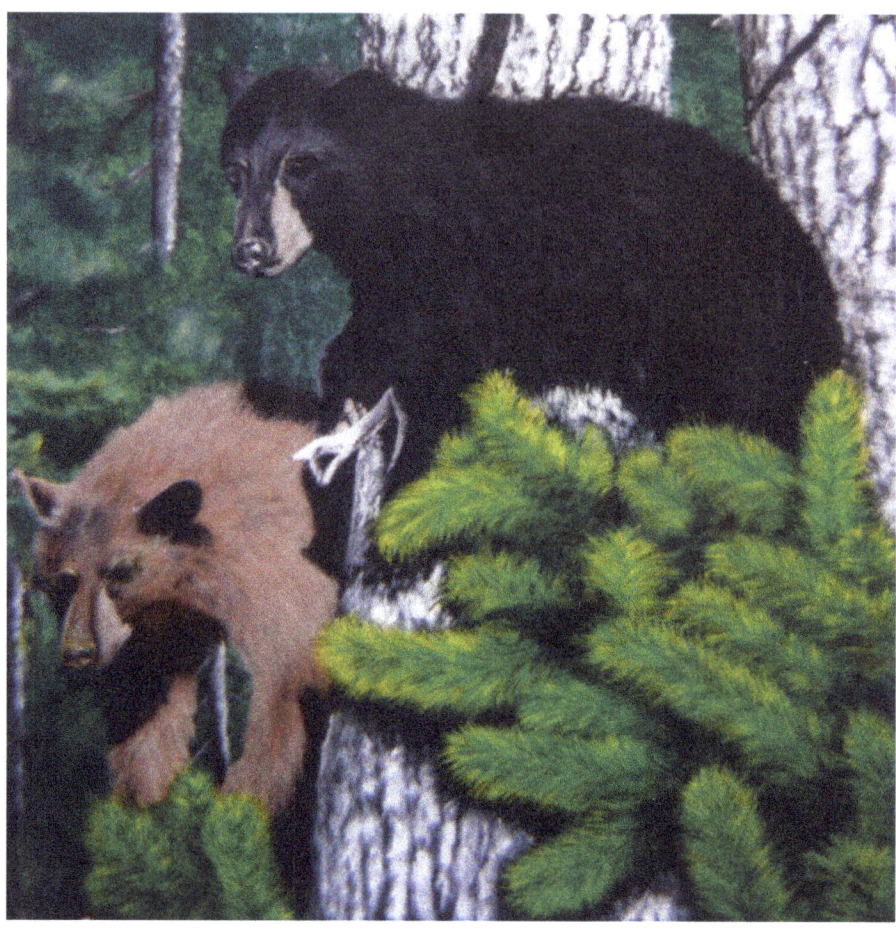

Bears

Bears can look cute and cuddly but again beware. Amongst the wild animals, other than the K-9 species bears are the closest thing to man's best friend, the domestic dog, which we have many. Quite often our bed and the couch are adorned by our four legged best friends. They literally sleep with us and think that is where they belong. We love our cuddly friends whether they are real or a foam-filled toy representation.

Bears, on the other hand are carnivores and they will eat you if given the opportunity. They are bigger than we are, have big claws, big teeth and the attitude and strength to use them. They hunt and forage to eat and feed their young. Respect is mandatory.

I have met them on several occasions; here is the story of one of those encounters. He was a black bear, which matched its description in all aspects.

He was solid black through and through; I did not see any trace of brown, not even on his snout or face which is most common amongst black bears. I am guessing this specimen weighed in at approximately three hundred fifty to four hundred pounds. He had a very fluffy coat so it was hard to tell the actual size. I was driving my old nineteen seventy-eight one-ton camouflaged Chevy pickup on a mountain road to go hunting with my bow. I had a tag for bear and deer, so I could legally hunt ether. I was hunting more for deer rather than bear, one reason is you hardly ever see bear and there are deer everywhere.

I had only seen a few bears before this encounter. Glimpses really, they are there one minute and poof like a ghost gone the next. I approached a flat area, plateau like, on one of the local mountains called Sawmill. There is a small campground at this location where the Angeles Crest trail passes through it. People are quite common in this area of the national forest, it is a great place for hiking, riding dirt bikes, camping and hunting.

Rolling slowly down the dirt road, out of nowhere, comes this big black fur ball running towards me on the road. I brought my camouflaged beast to a halt, stepped out of the truck bow in hand and knocked an arrow. The truck was still running with the door wide open, I was standing behind the door so I could hide my outline. I was ready! At approximately twenty yards, the brute hung a right and was trotting broadside to me. A perfect set up. I could not miss. Drawing my bow and pulling back the arrow I aimed, then hesitated as I admired this awesome creature. I had not planned to eat it, so I lowered my bow and watched it disappear into the wilderness, leaving a clear memory that has never faded. I have never bear hunted since.

We support our fish and game department when we purchase hunting or fishing licenses. Good healthy management of our wildlife is important and having the work force to protect it proves beneficial to us all. This means go buy a license of some sort and get out there and see what good management does for our environment. The wildlife is abundant here and we are fortunate to be able to see these majestic critters in the wild. I want to say "Thank you", to all those who risk their lives to protect our natural resources. Keep up the good work. I hope that our ancestors will have a green and healthy planet full of wildlife.

Here is another experience worth mentioning with our beloved friend, the bear. I had just moved into my newly purchased home which set on the edge of thousands of miles of national forest. My dog, Burbank, loved to sleep at the foot of my bed. At the time, he was about four months old and full of himself. It was peaceful and serene there with crickets chirping and not another sound, so sleeping was easy. Suddenly, Burbank was up barking frantically and wanting to protect me from the monster. The outside motion detector light came on and lit up the driveway below. I sat up and looked out the window just in time to see the big fat fluffy rear-end of a black bear just lumbering down my driveway. It was an easy walk from my water tank to the road, about eight hundred feet, and was apparently the main thoroughfare for the bear, connecting one side of the canyon to the other.

My first thought was, cool, I just saw my first bear. However, the next morning when I went out to tend to the chickens I saw all the damage the bear had done. First, I see my wooden outdoor patio table, the round kind, all smashed up and lying on the ground. I am thinking this must have been the noise that, my dog, Burbank heard that woke him up during the night. I never heard a thing. When I got to the chicken coup, I found two broken windows and the screen with three big claw marks cut through in an attempt to gain access. My mind starts racing and I am thinking the house could be next, or worse, it could be me! What I need is a fence that will keep a bear out.

Broke and barely able to pay the bills, I could not afford a new fence, so I got creative and bought used fencing and recycled. I made gates and fence posts using a combination of mostly used and recycled materials and a few new parts to create my safe zone from the beasts of the forest. I made it from chain link, wrought iron and natural stone. That way I could enjoy the way it looked and still see through it to enjoy the beauty of my surroundings, free from the dangers that lurked nearby, or so I thought. It turned out it was my human neighbors that were the ones to beware.

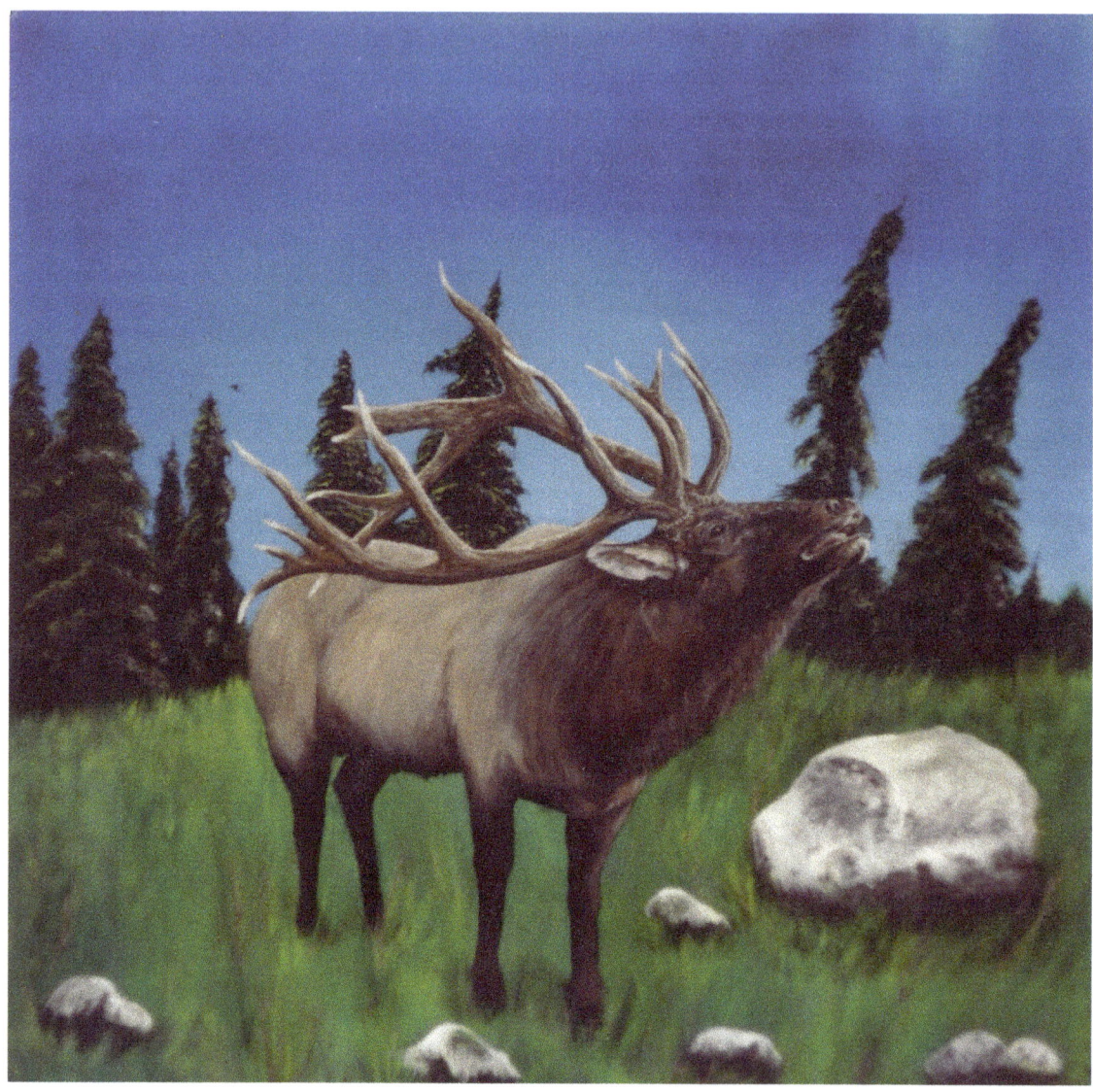

Elk

The majestic Elk is a magnificent creature, which has several different species such as the Tule Elk, Rocky Mountain Elk and the European Red Deer. This great creature can reach up to weights from six hundred to eleven hundred pounds and for the big males there, antlers can reach heights of four feet. The Rocky Mountain Elk is the most popular and abundant of the three in North America.

In many protected forests these majestic creatures reign as prince, their calls bugling out through mountain canyons like lonely spirits moaning for company, which is exactly what is happening during the fall, as the bulls call out for their perspective mates.

This animal is one of the most admired of the herbivores. I have been toe to toe and neck to neck with a few, lucky me. Unfortunately, they were behind a fence close to my mothers' house in Minnesota. The neighbors raise them for food. The elk's antlers are harvested and sold for furniture, chandeliers, jewelry and other items, in addition to being used as an aphrodisiac. Nothing goes to waste. Getting close to these somewhat tame animals is a treat.

Nature has a very delicate balance that must be preserved. If you cut down the forest, you destroy vital resources for life. We are getting better about select cutting and needless deforestation as well as needless killing. We are learning by our experiences that our very existence depends on taking care of our earth and its inhabitants. Just as we try to control animal populations to maintain a healthy order, we need to think about our own population as well. Our natural resources with our expanding population are being depleted. To maintain an equal balance of all living things and natural resources we must start showing more responsibility to this delicate eco system.

Moose

The moose is the largest of all the deer family (Cervidae), weighing between nine hundred and fourteen hundred pounds. Their antlers are on record; measuring up to eighty-one inches and can weigh as much as seventy pounds. They do not range, as far south as the Elk; the Moose is more of a northern native. They inhabit most of Canada and the colder regions of the USA. The Moose likes the water and they usually are found around wet areas eating its favorite foods. Their summer diet includes water lilies, willows and other aquatic vegetation. In the winter, they browse on twigs, buds and the bark of various other trees like Balsam, Dog Wood, Cherry, Aspen, Birch and Maple. When grazing these giants look totally calm and docile even approachable but beware these big beasts they will charge you and they are capable of speeds up to thirty-five miles an hour.

They can be very dangerous especially a mother with her calf, their protective nature can make them a lethal weapon. Urban sprawl keeps spreading into their habitat, thus making close encounters more prevalent. It is not uncommon in the great white north of the US and Canada to see one in your yard dining on, to them what seems to be a buffet of yummy treats, unaware that it is your prize flower garden.

I guess since you built your house in there back yard they have to collect the rent some how and since money has no meaning to them your garden will do just fine. I have never encountered a moose; I am looking forward to the possibility of that encounter.

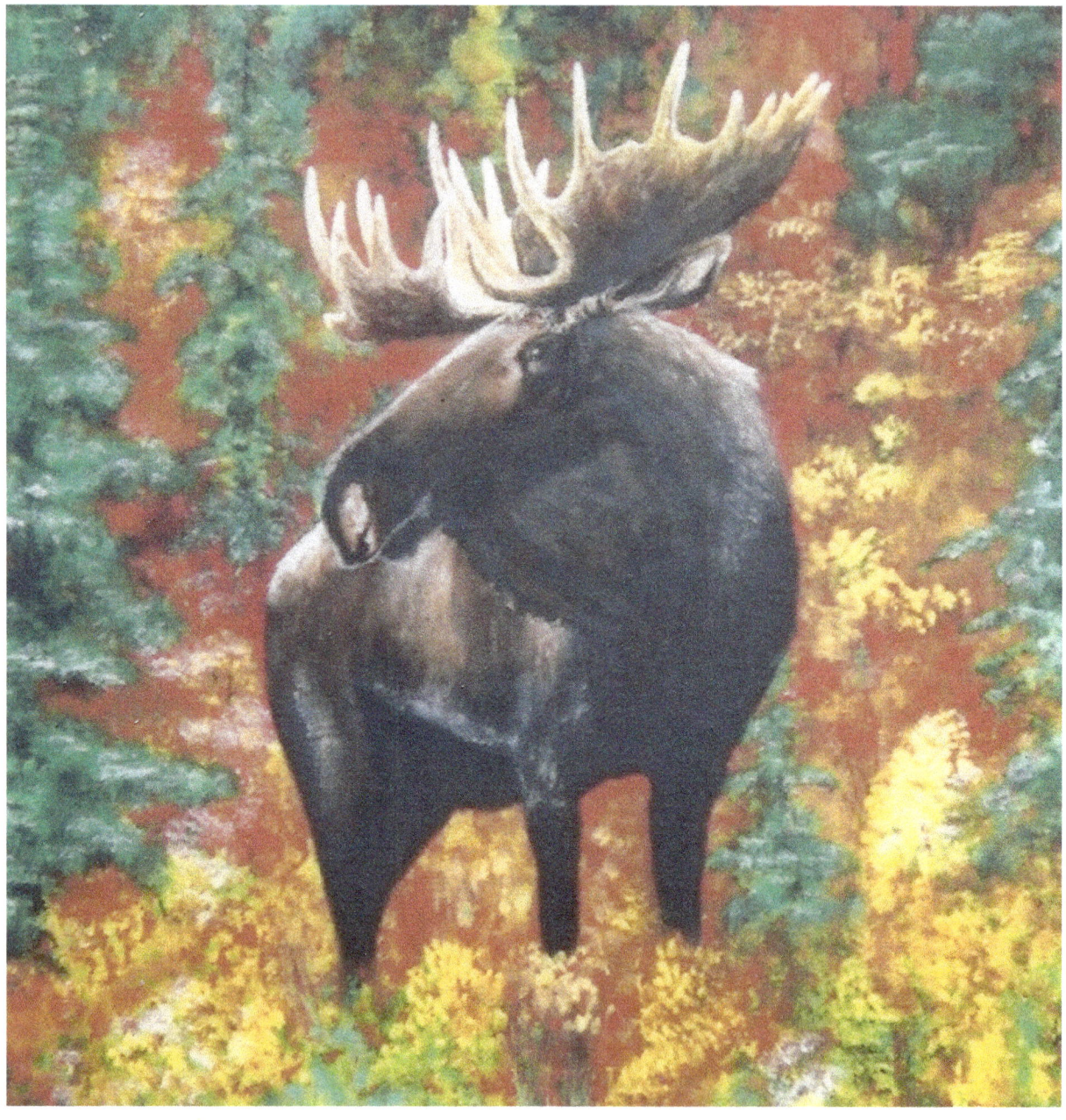

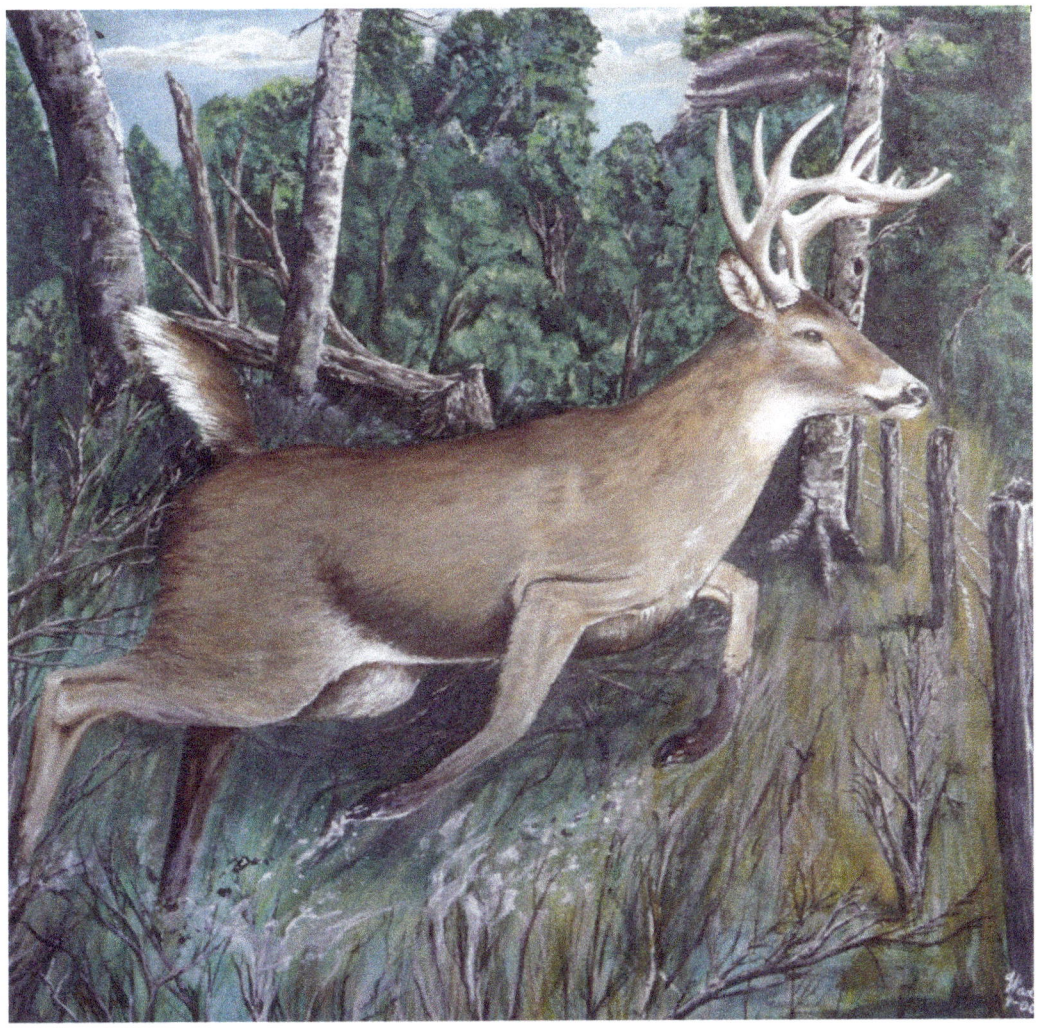

White Tail Deer

South Eastern Minnesota, is well known by many a hunter for its massive white tail deer. This impressive deer's antlers can spread in widths of approximately three feet. They can run up to thirty-five miles per hour and leap bounds of twenty feet. I have seen them jump the barbed wire fences of the fertile farmlands in the Midwestern U.S. They are elegant in their movements, like a ballet dancer.

Being from the area, I have seen many big bucks and I believe that there are world records held there for the size of their antlers. Also probably for their weight too, which can reach up to four hundred pounds. Houston Minnesota is home to many of my kin. One of whom owns Peterson taxidermy. Every time I visit, I make it a point to stop in and see all the trophy antlers and mounts of all the different animals. Taxidermy is an art form so I can relate to it. A good taxidermist can make these creatures look alive. It is a lot easier to draw or paint a picture of one when it is not moving. A deer in the wild will rarely stand still long enough to be photographed.

I love to watch them and all other animals of course. Wow, as I was writing this, I just caught a Grey Fox on video camera. One of the perks of writing in the woods, I find it much more rewarding than the confinement of an office or writing room. The wild animals large or small get my heart beating faster every time I get to see them.

I love the forest and go there every chance I get. When you sit, stand or lie down, "it really doesn't matter", just be still and quiet you may see all kinds of wild life. It is very peaceful for the most part. However, every living thing has to eat and the predators are lurking, looking for an easy meal. So take care as you venture quietly into the forest, you never know what you will see or what will see you.

Mule Deer

More stocky and muscular than the White Tail a Mule deer is built for the rugged terrain it inhabits. I have seen them climb a cliff in seconds, unlike the good hour it would take an experienced climber with his climbing gear. They too have very impressive antlers that can reach sizes of four feet in width, with their body weight up to four hundred and seventy five pounds.

I have seen many types of Mule deer. There are Desert Mule Deer, Columbian Black Tail, Sitka Black Tail, California Mule Deer, Inyo Mule Deer, and Rocky Mountain Mule Deer and maybe more I have not yet seen or heard of. I have noticed as the climates vary, a difference in their sizes occurs, the colder the climate the larger the deer seem to be.

For example, my wife and I visited Mazatlan Mexico; we went for a hike through the mountain trails where we came upon an enclosure, which housed some native deer, one of which was a seven-year-old buck. This mature, fully-grown deer probably weighed in at about forty pounds and his antlers only a spike no more than five inches tall. That is quite a size difference from the northern species I am used to seeing.

I have also noticed that deer in captivity are smaller than their wild counterparts. I truly do not believe there have been too many people that have been lucky enough to have seen an albino mule deer in the in the wild.

Well, I have seen one and have a photograph to prove it. I must say on that day, I did not take the picture. A couple of days later while driving home from town a friend also saw her and got a good picture before she disappeared into the brush. She was standing so perfectly still when I saw her. At first I thought, how did they build a snow deer with those spindly legs? Then I realized it was a real animal, a pure white mule deer. That is a rare sight and I feel extremely lucky to have seen her. Though I doubt she lived a long life. I have heard that the mother will run their white young off because they are so dissimilar, making them a target for predators. She was alone, left without the protection of the heard. No one that I know of has seen her since.

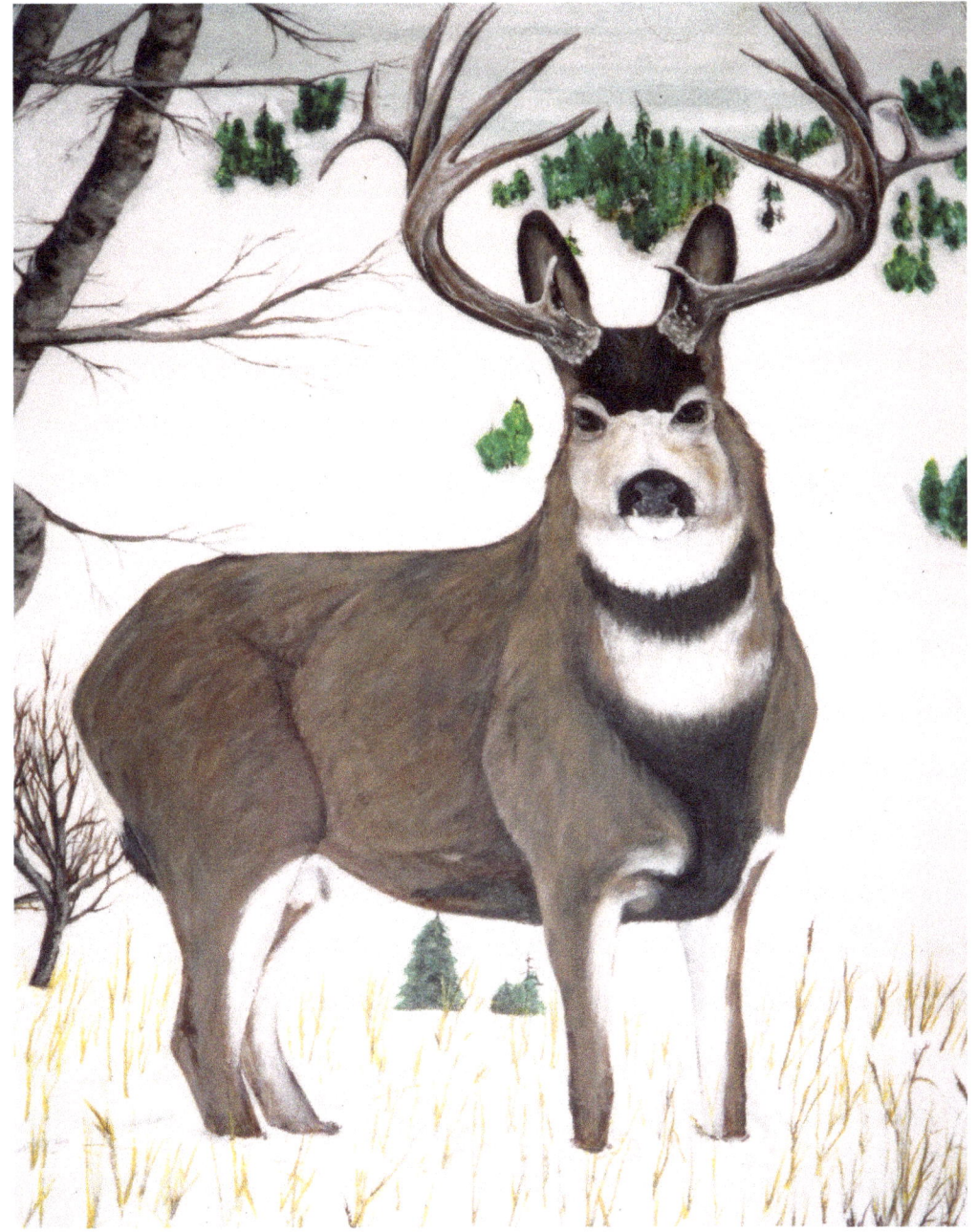

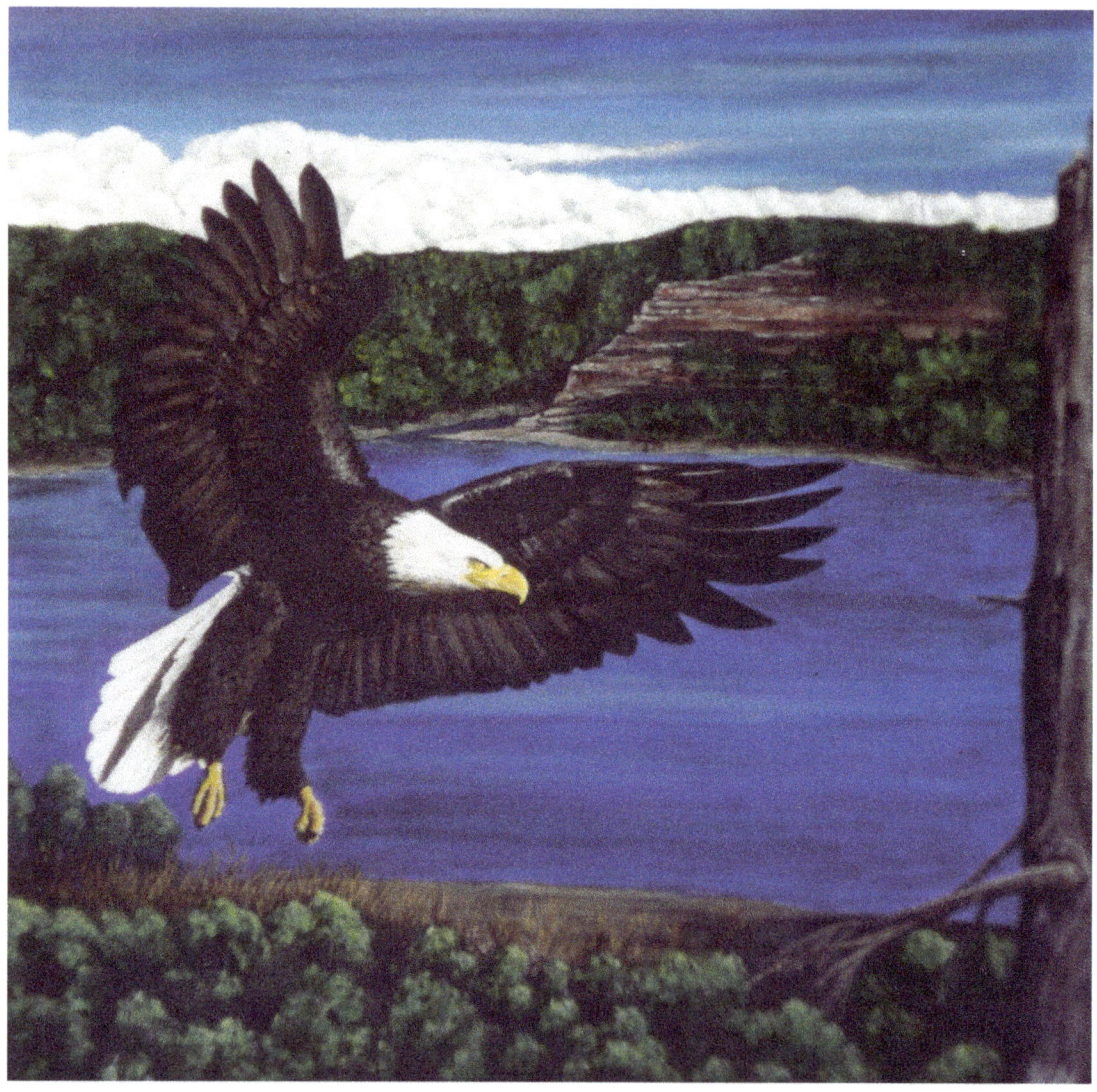

The Bald Eagle

In my early twenties when I still lived in South Eastern, Minnesota, I was working for a local tree trimming company our job was to keep the lines clear for the power company. One cold and clear day, mid-winter, I was about half a mile up a hill covered with three to four feet of snow to take off one branch on a monster oak tree. The hardest part was getting there carrying all that gear.

My supervisor sent me on this two to three hour journey so he could take a nap. He drank to much the night before, and was feeling the effects of his gluttony for alcohol. I did not mind, I was away from him for a while, a blessing in disguise. After what seemed like an hour, walking through deep snow, up hill, with a bunch of gear I finally reached the designated tree. After resting a bit, I climbed the monster. I positioned myself way up in a comfortable crotch, as comfortable as it gets for a tree anyway. Then I took a break and looked out over the Mississippi River Valley. Frozen over, the snow and ice making everywhere you looked bright white. It made my eyes hurt.

I was all tied in and ready for my task at hand staring out at the awesome view. When up from below me a bald eagle soars up to land right where I am in the tree and got within a few feet of me. His feet adorned with deadly talons reaching out to land on the branch where I was perched next too. This majestic bird and I made eye contact. His eyes bulged wide, probably just like mine, when he realized I was standing there. With a quick turn and flap of wings, I felt the rush of air on my face as he made this maneuver and was gone.

I have always dreamed of being able to fly like an eagle, even if just for a day. It would be so incredible to be able to fly high in the air and see the sites from above, unlimited by the confines of gravity. It seems to me that it would be the ultimate freedom. Well, maybe in another life I will get to be an eagle or a hawk or an owl. I guess any bird will do. Speaking of owls, here is a pair of paintings I did for a little old woman who loved owls.

Snowy Owl

I once had a run-in with a barn owl and this is an encounter I will never forget. It was shortly after sundown at my friend Scott's house in Southern California. His dog Buddy "a black German Sheppard mix" and I were walking out side of his house to dump some trash when Buddy suddenly dashed behind a trash can and came out with what I thought to be a white chicken. Scott did not have chickens. I yelled at Buddy to drop it and like the good dog he was, he immediately obeyed my command and came right over and sat at my feet. The chicken rolled to its back and spread its wings.

It was at that moment I realized this was not a chicken; my heartbeat went up a notch. This was a large owl with its feet sticking straight up at me, talons splayed out ready for battle. He hissed out this sound of warning as he repeatedly snapped at me with his razor sharp hooked bill. I stepped back to avoid being the victim of a pissed off owl and when I did this he just laid there for what seemed like a minute showing off his weapons of mass destruction.

With the agility of a cat, he spun around then quickly got to his feet, took a few steps and flew away without a sound. This to me is amazing for a bird of that size to be capable of flying without making as much as the slightest sound. Buddy and I looked at each other and smiled.

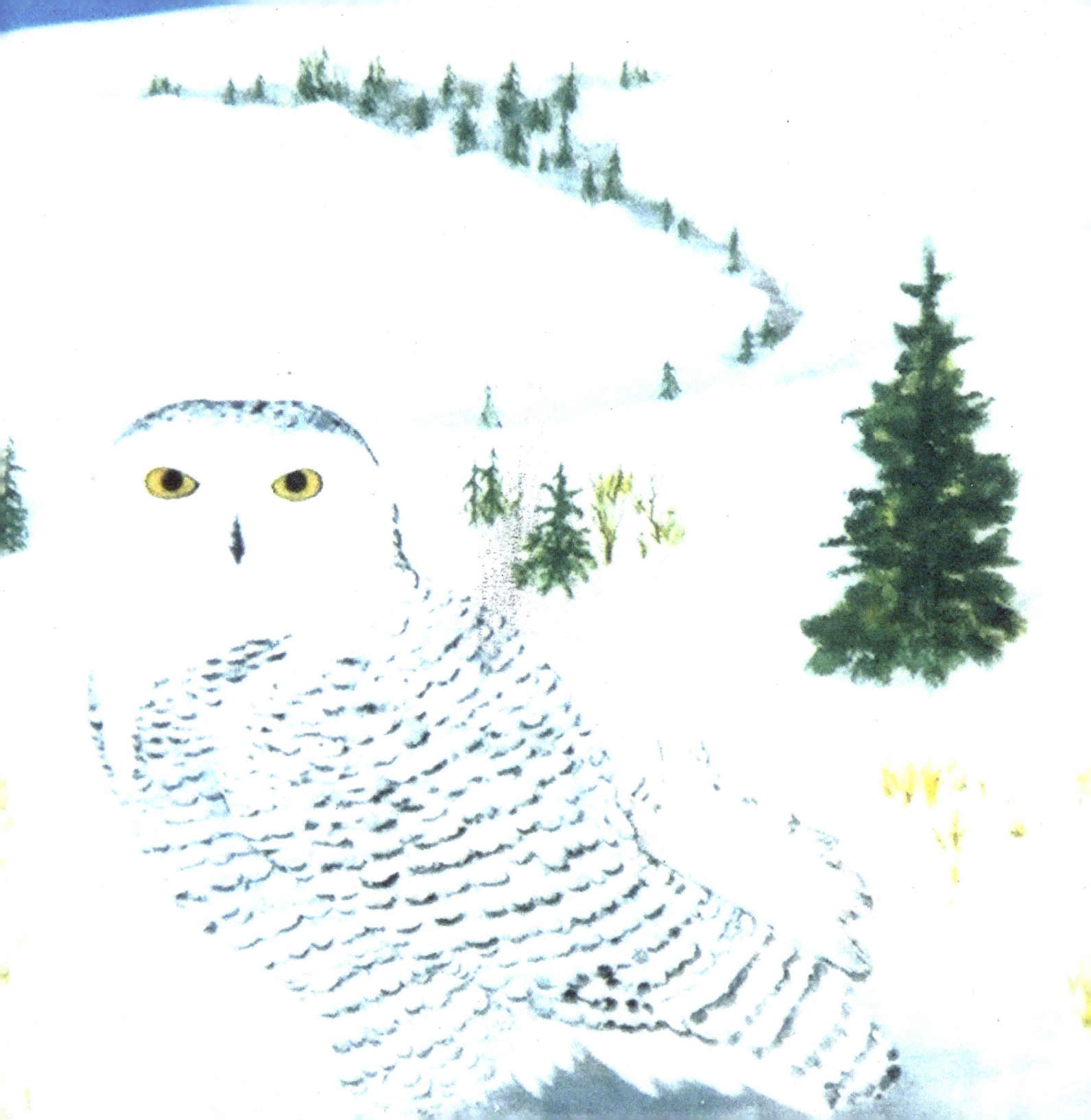

On another occasion, I was sitting in a blind that I made out of sticks and branches from the woods around me. This made it easier for me to move around without scaring the critters. It was just before sunrise and the sky was just beginning to lighten. The Eastern sky had turned pink as the sun was approaching the earth's horizon.

I saw what appeared to be an owl land in a tree about twenty yards to my right. Always interested I strained to see what it was when it flew to a closer tree and landed. When I watched it fly in silence, I knew it was an owl. Then it flew even closer again landing in another tree, and yet again until it was right at eye to eye level with me just within arms reach. It just sat there looking at me. This little bird was a pigmy owl not much bigger than my hand. This little owl was as interested in me as I was in it. We were checking each other out for a couple of minutes, when I found it to hard to resist the temptation to touch the creature that was analyzing me in such a way. Therefore, without fear I reached up exposing the back of my hand with hopes of him perching on it and off the little fellow flew.

I suppose with me making a move he figured it out that I was in fact alive. These kinds of experiences are what keep me drawn to nature; they are rare and treasured occasions for me indeed.

Great Horned Owl

This is not a picture of the little pigmy, however I thought you might like to see it. This big bird is a Great Horned Owl.

I have always wondered why it is, that the critters get so close to me, it is as if they are unafraid. Once while I was in Mexico some friends and I were sitting around the campfire, all of a sudden a kangaroo rat wanted to climb up in my lap. No kidding it come right to me, gets on my shoe and starts climbing up. I kicked out with a flick and flung it a few feet away. I thought there might be something wrong with it like rabies, and to my surprise it came right back. Up my leg it went. I got the willies and I am not to macho to tell you goose bumps covered my body. I jumped up and kick flicked him off me again, this time the little fellow flew a little farther and did not come back, thankfully. Another rodent that likes to check me out when I am out in the woods are squirrels, many have come right up to me to see what I am. I have even had them climb over me when I have been sitting quiet and still. I have come to expect it to happen and it does. One time even a raccoon walked up to me and was about to climb up my leg. Sorry, but that time I had to poke her and tell her no. She scurried off in a hurry when she realized I was a human, I guess I looked like a tree. I do not see how she could have made such a mistake, but for some reason known only to her, I was something to climb.

By the way, I know it was a she because she had one toddler with her. I have had many close encounters with the wildlife, I am sure I do not remember them all. On several occasions, I have also had humming birds land on my finger when they needed a place to rest.

All of these experiences have led me to believe I am "One With Nature".

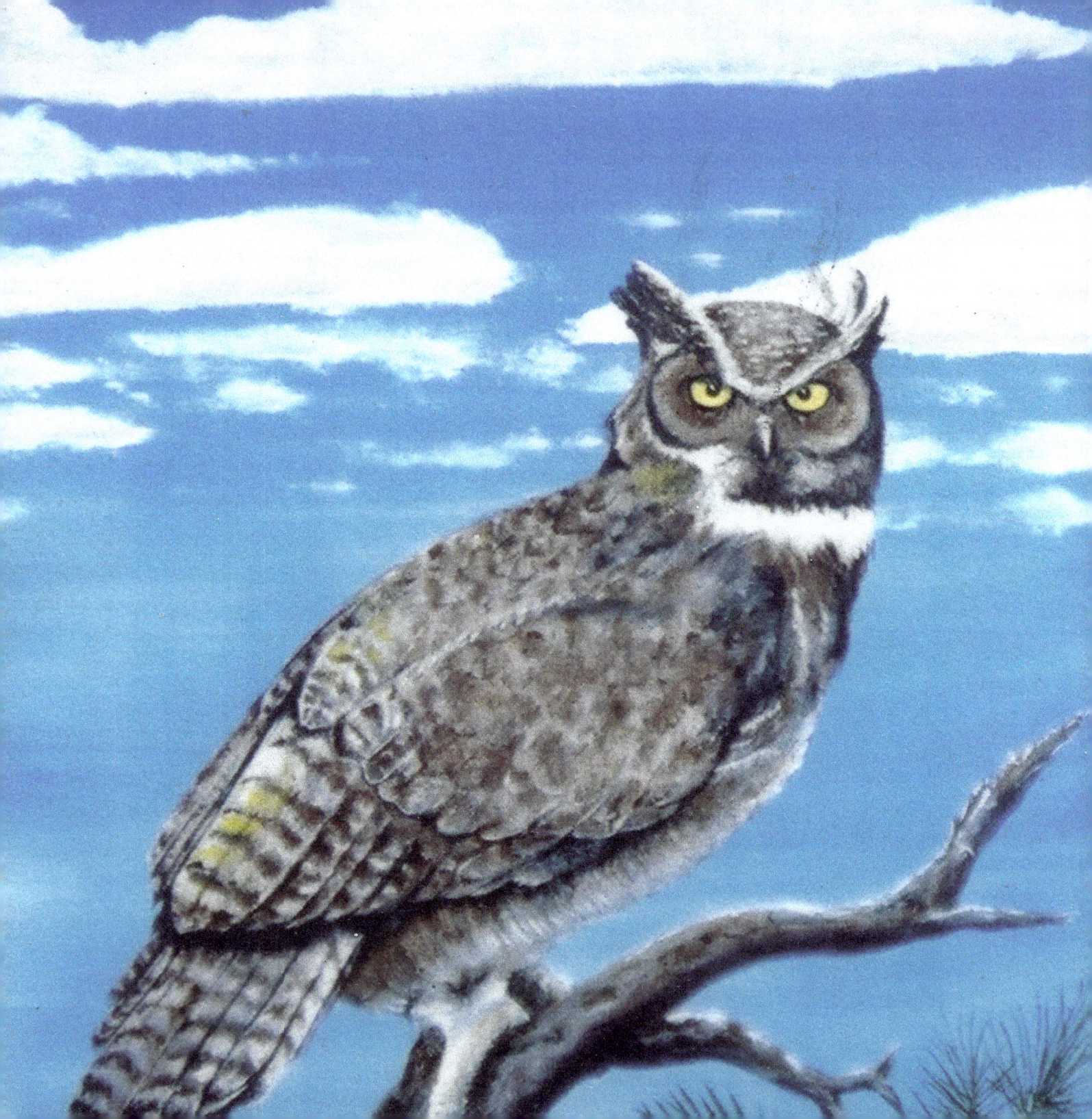

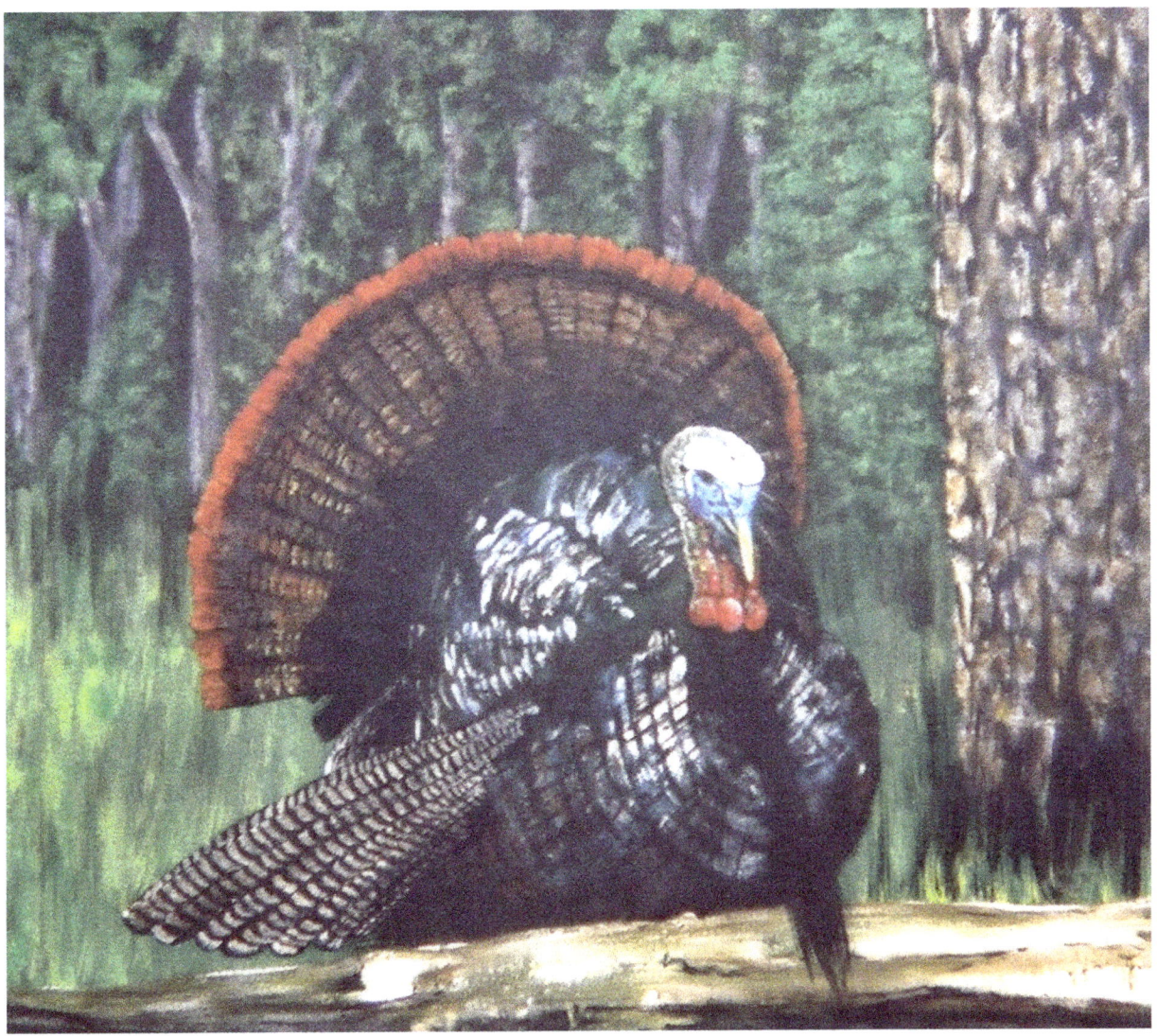

The Elusive Wild Turkey

The wild Turkey is native to North America and our domestic versions although white in color are of the same species. Adult toms (males) normally weigh between eleven to twenty four pounds. However, the record weight for an adult male is thirty-eight pounds. Females (hens) are much smaller averaging between six to twelve pounds. Subspecies include the Eastern, Osceola,

Rio Grand, Merriam's, Gould's and the South Mexican wild turkey.

According to a letter written to his daughter Sarah, Benjamin Franklin would have preferred the wild turkey to the Bald Eagle for our National bird. He thought the Bald Eagle to be of bad moral character, lazy, cowardly and did not make his living honestly. The Bald Eagle often steals from other animals who have diligently procured their meal. To him the honest and brave turkey would have been a much better choice.

In the mass population growth of the Wild West, during the gold rush, the turkey was chosen as a food source for its protein by the pioneers. Early settlers preferred the turkey do to their ability to survive on the scant food supply and their ease in over coming obstacles.

There is a small valley in Southeastern Minnesota lined with hardwood trees, oaks, hickory, walnut and the like. Groves of tall Birch trees dot the hillsides adding white to the multitude of fall colors that paint the landscape in October. Apple trees of different types mixed intermittently amongst the thick under growth of wild black berry bushes and sumac. Left unattended they are the remnants of a long forgotten orchard. Rows of Pine trees planted long ago for Christmas harvest line the hillside opposite the tan farmhouse. The barn and other out buildings are all painted red with white trim.

A small stream runs through the valley, clean and clear full of small Brook trout, eventually spilling into a larger creek, which in turn runs into a river. The flat bottoms of the valley are cultivated for the black soil is rich in nutrients. Rotating crops such as Corn, Soybeans and Alfalfa yearly helps the soil to not become depleted if its nutrients.

This is one of many paradises, my cousin Jared is lucky enough to call this one home. There are literally hoards of wild turkey that inhabit the area. Every evening about an hour before sunset, groups of sometimes thirty or more come out of the woods to forage in the open fields for food. Deer will often accompany these hungry fowl during the feeding hours, using their extra eyes as sentries to warn them of approaching danger. Jared works hard every year planting food plots for the wild animals, consisting of turnips, pumpkins, corn and winter greens, making this a very much needed and appreciated buffet for all the wild life to enjoy.

Like most outdoorsmen, he is ever a conservationist. Much thanks to him and all the others that do the same in their effort to help preserve our forests and animals for generations to come.

Toucan Bird

Birds, exotic and colorful, are by far the most beautiful of all the species of animals in my opinion; with their vast array of types and color combinations birds are stunning. For the painter of wildlife, the multitude of choices will leave the artist with many creative avenues for selection. I have only painted a few birds. The head shot of a male Toucan is one of my favorites. It has a 3D look in the eye that is hard to create.

The Toucan is native to Tropical America and is a fruit eater. A common belief is that birds are dinosaurs that have evolved over millions of years to adapt to the current conditions on earth at this time. I believe the fossil record proves this and it looks like we, as humans will in the near future be able to trigger the right genetic sequence and have dinosaurs back from the past. Not that this is such a good idea do not forget Jurassic Park.

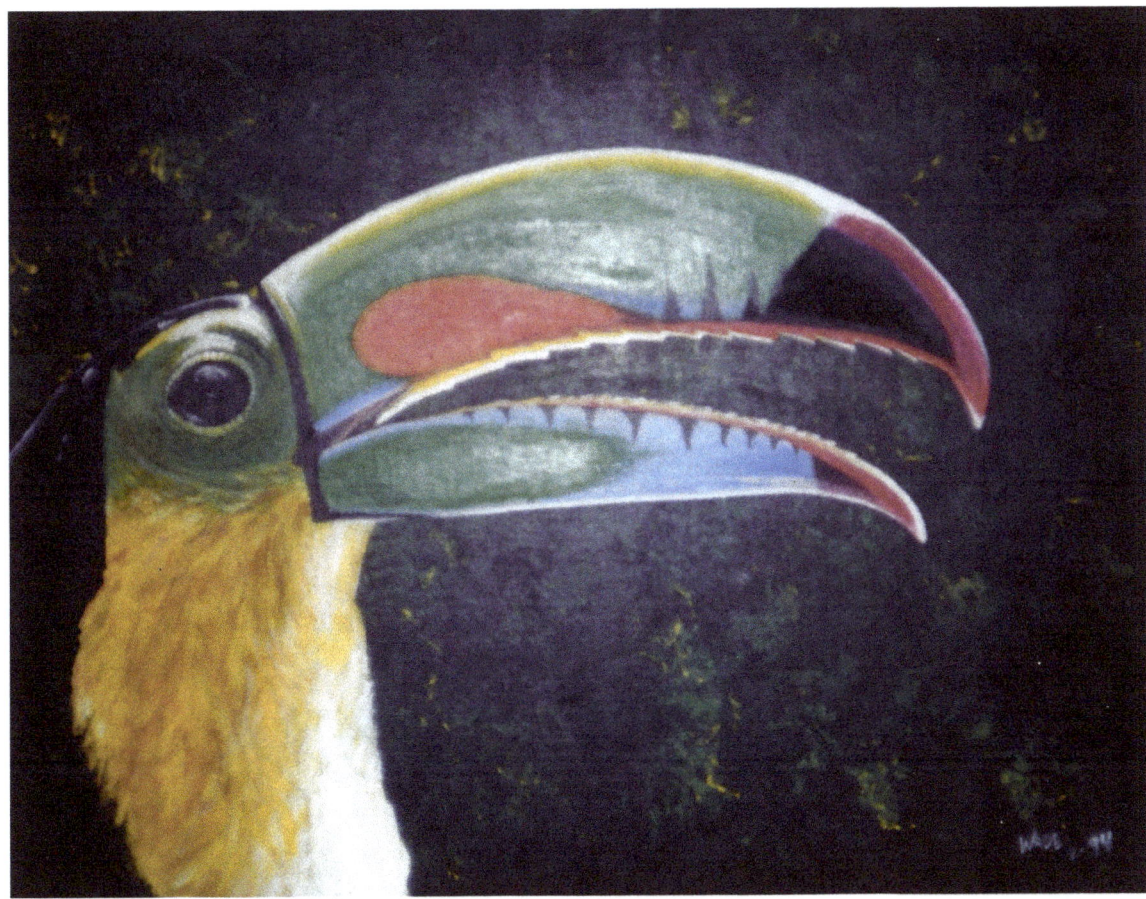

I believe in safety first, probably from being in construction for the better part of my life. Something always seems to go wrong. For example, my 9th grade geography teacher lived right above us when I was in high school in an area called, Pleasant Ridge.

He farmed on the side, had some acreage and did all the work himself. One summer evening he was out in the fields bailing hay and did not come home at his usual time. So his wife went out looking for him only to come up on his tractor and hay bailer still running but her husband was no where to be found . She called the police and an investigation ensued. After hours of searching the woods and the surrounding areas, they finally found him in the hay bailer. It seems some how he managed to get caught in the raking part that picks with the hay with spring loaded steel forks. Three cylinder shaped rows of them, rotating opposite each other to pick up the dried hay and feed it into an opening that leads to chopping blades that cut and fold the hay then ties them into bails.

Poor Guy that had to be an awful way to go. This is akin to being eaten alive only by your own tools for making a living. Your body goes into shock when exposed to extreme trauma and you do not feel the pain. I guess this is one thing that some of us will only experience once.

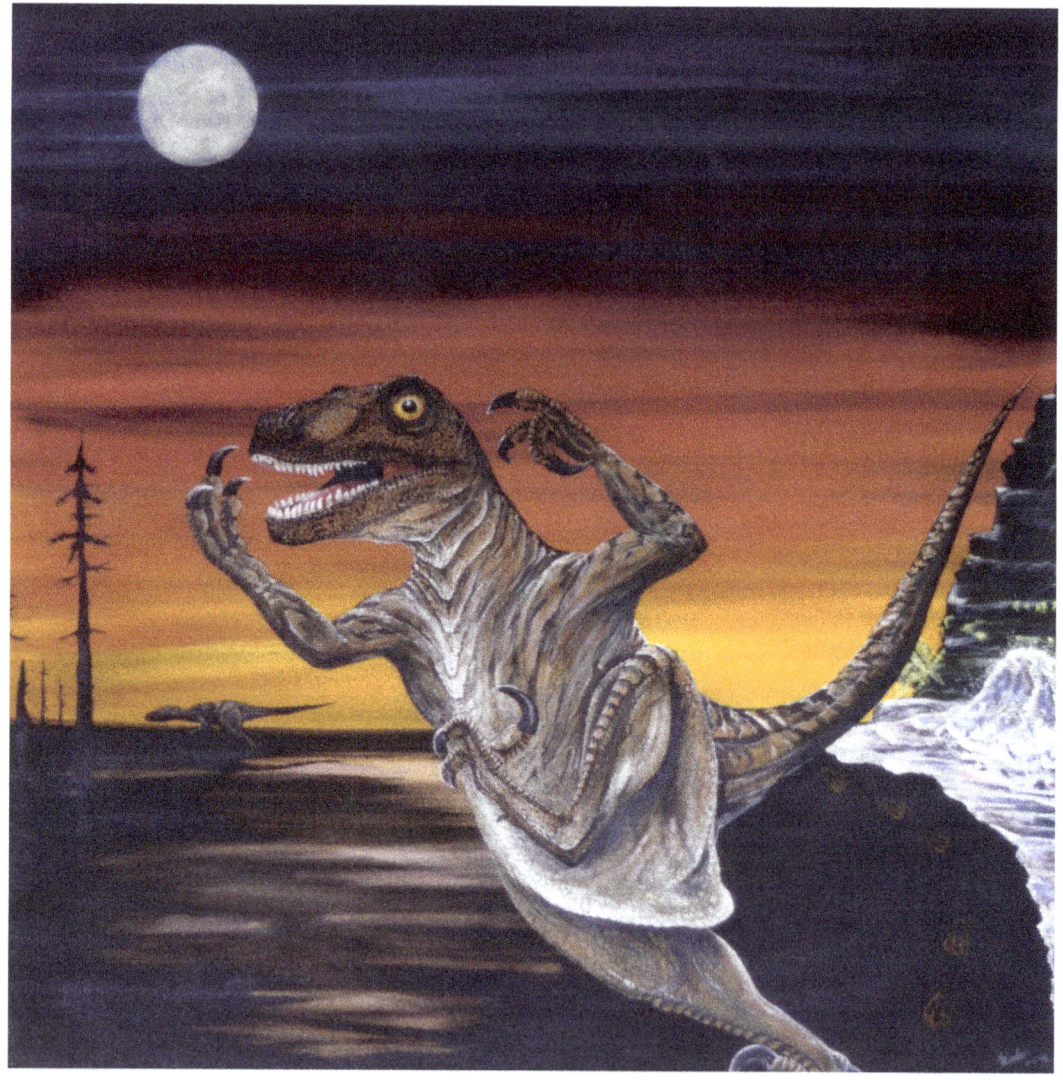

Deinonychus

Deinonychus was a raptor dinosaur, which was approximately six feet tall and weighed about the same as full grown man. They were in the Dromaeosaurid family of dinosaurs. Dromaeosaurid mean "swift reptile". They had a large six-inch sickle-shaped claw that could rotate one hundred eighty degrees; they used this for slicing into their prey. These ferocious and terrifying creatures ate many of their victims alive. Thankfully, they are now extinct.

Man the predator

I am a predator, a killer. I hunt other life forms to feed my hunger, mammals, birds, reptiles, amphibians, insects and plants. I am an omnivore. Like the bear, I will consume almost anything to survive. I am the dominant animal, more intelligent and more capable with my agile hands. I have long legs for sustained travel and pursuit. I can run down most of my prey or out last them in a drawn out hunt. I can outsmart them and use tools to get them easier, and have forward facing eyes for binocular vision. I can capture and farm them for slaughter at a later date. I am human. Like you, I hunt and gather, but unlike the majority of you, most of my food comes from the wild. Not from farms that use growth hormones, antibiotics, herbicides, pesticides and fungicides. There are probably more harmful agents that I could list, but I just do not know about them.

The food that nature provides me with is pretty much poison free, I feel like it is my very own Garden of Eden. Our Mother Earth provides, I never take more than I need and give back all I can. By thinking of your surroundings as a gift, you can achieve harmony with our Mother (nature). Most humans hunt at the grocery store, but there are still those of us that follow the ways of ancient man, trying to stay as true to our ancestry as modern civilization will allow. However, let it be said we all are predators whether you hunt at the market or hunt in the woods, you are a killer. Directly or indirectly, your actions cause the death of other life forms. Embrace it, except it, because of our ancestry we are who we are and smarter because of it.

Our brains grew larger because of eating proteins instead of just plant material. Making us the creative thinkers, we are today. Our advances in technology are a good example of our brilliance. We are capable of much more. We have the ability to imagine and create. Now if we could only get this brutal predator, 'human' to use their brilliance for good instead of destruction, humans might come out of this with a clean and healthy earth for our offspring to enjoy for millions of more years.

Lucky Dog

Have you ever met a rattlesnake eye-to-eye, head up hissing, and ready to strike? Luckily, I have never been bitten, but that is not the case with a dog I once had. `Buster, my twelve year old chocolate lab, red Doberman mix met up with a rattler one day. He was one hundred pounds of sheer love and spry as a puppy. Brave and strong, full of energy and smart as any dog I have ever met. His curiosity would get him in trouble at times though. I am sure he probably saved me from a snakebite by finding the snake in my house first.

With no experience with snakes, Buster must have approached the snake in the usual curious doggy way, with his nose sniffing and poking at the snake. I am sure the rattler wasted no time striking out in defense. Luckily, for Buster, his fang only penetrated one nostril. When I found him, he was sitting in the doorway to my bedroom. His face was so proliferated I almost did not recognize him. His head looked like a balloon, swollen to almost twice its size and his chest starting to swell as well. I rushed him to the emergency room for in hopes that he could receive antivenin in time.

They administered the medicine and gave him a good prognosis, the doctors took real good care of him and after a couple of days he was back as good as ever, except for the pupil in his left eye. The pupil was permanently dilated, leaving him sensitive to light. During day light, he would keep that eye closed. Buster lived sixteen years, considered a long life for a large breed. We were best friends and I enjoyed the many miles we shared together walking on this earth.

I lived in the Pine Canyon house for about five years. During that time there were many times I had to dispense of rattlesnakes, both inside and out. It took me awhile to find and fix all the holes and access points to stop the snakes from entering the house. By using good common sense we can coexist with our neighbors, mine being critters of every kind, without doing unnecessary harm. You can watch rattle snakes, but do not touch them. They are not the touch me type if you know what I mean.

These reptiles are a necessary part of our ecosystem as they help to control the rodent populations. Again, these animals are to be respected and appreciated for what they are capable of and what they do. If my wife is on the road and sees one trying to get across, to see that it achieves its goal unharmed, she will actually pullover and help it to the other side. I have often wondered how she knows which side of the road the snake wants to be on? She is a brave woman and has a true connection to the animals. She is like the Dog Whisperer and the Horse Whisperer all rolled into one. She is a regular Dr. Doolittle and she has that sixth sense for animals. She knows what the animals want just by looking into their eyes, she says it is just a feeling that comes over her and their needs become clear.

Now mind you, if the animal does not want the help, she will not push it. The thing is if it is in their best interest, she can usually talk them into co-operating with her. I am amazed and impressed by her ability to tame the beast within these critters. A Mother of Nature in her own right. She has saved the lives of many animals including snakes with or without rattles. If she could she would save all the critters, except maybe a tasty trout or crappie but even with those, she has been known to fight for their right to live.

Fish are a big part of our diet though, so it is usually only for the smaller ones that she feels have not had the chance to live their lives yet. We as humans need fish in our diets. As we, all know the fish live in water; it does not take a genius to figure that one out. So by polluting your or anybody else's water you pollute the food we consume not to mention turn the natural beauty of our outdoors into a unsightly mess. It is all of ours to enjoy. Keep it clean and pristine. That means if you pack it in; then pack it out and recycle your waste.

Oh yeah, no graffiti please. It does not belong in the forest on nature's canvas, if you like to paint so much go paint your mother's house and maybe the neighbors will see what a good job you did and maybe give you a job because of it. Then you will not have time to paint the rocks with your ignorant territorial claims. You will actually do something useful in life instead of being destructive. I was remembering a walk up a canyon along a clean, clear perfect stream to a waterfall in the forest with a nice pond for swimming. It was so beautiful except for the graffiti. How lame is it to ruin that beautiful scene, created for all of us to enjoy and defile it with spray paint. Of course, this does not apply to all that are reading this, but for those it does apply to you know who you are, I hope this makes you think about what you are doing and stop.

Water World

Our Earth's surface is two-thirds water; it is the life giver to all that lives, and without it, all life dies. Look at Mars; it is a perfect example; no water, no life. We know life can exist in extreme heat and cold. Life can and does exist all over the universe. However, we do not live there, we live here. This is our own aquarium, our earth. Like your aquarium with your pet frog in it, if the water dries up, so does your frog. Ancient civilizations worshipped water, and for good reason. A bad drought would wipe them out and they knew that. We only have a limited supply of water and it is getting to the point where that supply is diminishing. With the Earths population growing out of control, what little supply we have left is being used up fast, forcing us to use treated water to water our fields and live stock and yes our public as well. How many times do you think we can retreat our already retreated water? Too many people, excess demands, equals limited supply. Do the math people. How many kids does one person need to have? I have known too many to have eight or more, that is too many. The earths population is now seven billion and rising.

A little self-control and common sense please. Perhaps the fertility doctors should be a little more concerned for all of our well-beings too, opposed to their own financial well-being. In my opinion they have gotten way out of control, woman are having litters instead of a baby.

"Wade in the water, Wade in the water", a very old chant my fellow peers in grade school used to chime out to me with glee, as they teased me about my name. Now I think they were jealous because I had a cool name, either way, I have been wading in the water since I was a baby, so it fits me to a tee. I am the only member of my immediate family to be able to swim. I learned by watching other people swim. I copied them and viola, it worked. I could swim with no formal training at about five years old. My life as well as all life forms is based in and around water. Water should be worshipped. I am proud to bear the name of Wade, in the water.

Success in life to me is not in the monetary thing. I have never strived to be wealthy, only to be happy and proud of my accomplishments. I do everything to the best of my capabilities, I try to achieve my goals and be one with my environment. In being that way, I have no guilt about anything I have done so I am at peace with myself. I hope my words will inform others to be that way. I am fortunate to have learned to live this life style; I did so by listening to the great teacher Mother Nature. She speaks with wisdom and if you take the time to listen you will hear her too. Hug your trees for they give you life through the fruit that they bare and the oxygen they produce and the carbon dioxide they consume. Try planting a tree or two and experience the joy of watching them grow, reap the rewards that Mother Nature has to offer, and apple pie is not bad either.

Communication with all

Some believe when you talk to your plants they respond and grow better, I for one believe this is true. Like all things living, plants need love too. With the care that comes from love, the plant receives water regularly, is dusted off when needed and even the carbon dioxide it gets when you talk to it, are all the things needed for its life to flourish and it shows a visible response. In return, the plant gives back food, oxygen, beauty and medicinal uses, not to mention the simple pleasures we get from growing them.

All life is connected and all life communicates with each other, non-verbally as well as verbally. Like with your dog as an example, he learns your words like sit, stay, lie down, come, go bye-bye, etc. You in return learn their certain barks, grunts, groans and other noises that make up their language. We also have the ability like our dogs and other animals to communicate telepathically however the majority of the human race has forgotten how to do so.

Take notice to your dog when you are thinking of going out somewhere observe how they act. My dogs get all exited and start begging to go with me, that is only one example, there are many more. Sometimes I truly believe they get into my head. They do not know how to tell time yet when my wife is on her way home from work still out of ear distance from home they get exited, her work schedule varies so I know they are not programmed.

I believe through, the love you share with them the bond between your animals creates a gift of unspoken communication. I have experienced it and seen it for myself with those I love, from having the same thoughts as my wife to telling my dog to come when he is out of my site. I run these little tests just to see if they will work, well they do. For example, I will tell one of my dogs to get over here in my mind and he comes running straight to me. This has happened to many times for it to be a coincidence. Sometime I will tell my big boy Red to get off the bed with only a thought and he complies; I will tell him to sit he does. My wife also does this with her dogs, it is the same for her, this happens all too often for it to be anything but telepathic communication. So I say coincidence, I think not.

I see these traits of animal communication in my wife just in the way they instinctively respond to her and treat her with respect and kindness, this includes even the mean ones and they usually do as she asks. It is almost comical to watch the way some of these critters suck up to her showering her with their affection, most treat her as their alpha. I truly believe she is one with nature, I know I have said it before but it really is something to see. In communicating, the list goes on with many forms of life. If you have a green thumb for instance maybe you are communicating with the plants and do not even know it, but they do. I know many other people feel this unspoken ability to communicate. I believe it is measured by the bond each individual person has with life. How fortunate the human race would be if we could use this ability to communicate with all life forms.

Like the movie Avatar, one with their entire planet and every thing in it. There would be no war or greed only harmony, peace and love. What a fantasy an Eden so to speak. Our earth is crying in pain from the balance being off, sort of like a person with disease or injury would. Maybe global warming is the communication; this could be an SOS, the cry for care and repair. Humanities disrespect will be met with horrific consequences if we as a whole do not change our belligerent disregard for the importance of the simple appreciation, care and understanding of our precious mother earth. The force of nature responds to our communication "I don't care, I'll take what I want and it doesn't matter" will be met with our certain demise.

Our eco system is fragile, depletion of our resources and not replenishing what we take, not maintaining the balance and using good management is arrogant and well just plain dumb considering we as a race have the knowledge to do other wise. Fishing out the oceans and over harvesting the forests etcetera is not maintaining the balance. This is bound to leave us with no water to drink, no air to breath and no food to eat. There you have it the end of life, as we know it. We are wasteful and greedy, finning sharks comes to mind, why waste the rest of the fish? This is wanton waist not to mention cruel. It sends a message to the earth and it is not a positive one. When you use her up and drain her dry you seal your own fate, she will have no more to give leaving us with no more to take.

Karma

I feel these sayings hold true. You get what you give, reap what you sow, you are what you eat and live by the sword die by the sword and so on. Therefore, if you go through life being a louse to others you will most likely be treated accordingly. When we use toxins to kill plants (weeds), bugs, fungus, we poison the earth, water and all that sustains us to live. If we make these things and distribute them into our environment we are consuming them as well, even if it's not intentional, either thru our skin, breathing the air, eating our farmed food and don't forget drinking the treated water. Even if you have a well that does not necessarily mean you are safe from toxic distribution. Toxins and poisons will seep into the aquifer too.

When we contract certain awful diseases or illnesses that toxins will inflict on us, caused by our own careless actions, we have only ourselves to blame or could that be karma at work? Being "One With Nature", means taking care of what has been given to us, not destroying the very things that keep us alive. In my opinion, creating nuclear weapons or nuclear power plants is completely irresponsible. This technology should not be used for any purpose, whether it is for electricity or destruction.

Just look at what happened to the victims of Three Mile Island in 1979 and the Chernobyl disaster in 1986 then there is the most recent in Japan 2011, leaving the Japanese city heavily contaminated and this is just to mention a few. Unless collectively we think our existence on this earth should become extinct, a change in our ways is mandatory.

I believe we as the earths superior beings have yet to learn to control our greed, lust for power, hatred, anger and all the other negative and destructive things we are capable of. Maybe we will destroy our selves before nature does. Only time will tell. This all could be avoided if society as a whole would come together to make the necessary changes that could help insure our survival. Show respect for mother earth and this will also help in upping our odds for the future of our and other species.

Every time I turn the news on or pick up the newspaper it reminds me of just how bad our world has become, our selfish greed for power and control is running rampant. People fighting and dying to take possession of something that was here long before us and will be here long after, these things like water, land, food, oil etc. were given to us all, as a gift. These things should be treated as such; instead, we treat them as our own personal possession. Greed and selfishness is an evil act that leads to the disrespect and the lack of appreciation for the gifts we have been blessed with.

Our actions will come back to us in one way or another, in this life and maybe in the next. I truly feel that way. If only all people felt this way we would have no war, no greed, no stealing, and no murder, none of the bad things that make up this life we all live in. The choices are ours. We as human beings can make it anyway we want. We have the intelligence and the physical capabilities to do anything.

We should start with ourselves. To better ourselves and to better our environment should be our main goal. If we want to continue to exist as a race, we must take care of our environment. Extinction is not an option for me.

Insects

As the human race, we can all pretty much agree on at least one thing, we hate bugs. We poison them on a regular basis with insecticides around the home, farm, business excreta, in doing so we put those poisons in our environment. We need to think this one over, is it to our advantage to poison our selves because of the dislike we have for bugs? Only recently have I noticed new products out there that take this bad habit in to consideration by making the bug killing products safer for all living things considered. When producing these products, we should be using biodegradable and nontoxic all natural substances to kill there intended target (the insect) leaving the environment and other living things to live unharmed. Thanks goes out to the creators of these new safer products. Maybe there is hope for humanity, after all.

The use of biodegradable and nontoxic products are being used by some, however if it does not turn into the majority I fear for the survival of all living things alike. Here is an alternate option to poisoning insects, take the locusts swarms for example, we should harvest the manna from heaven. Catch them, cook or dry them and feed them to farmed fish or chickens, turkeys, pigs and the list could go on, in the uses they could be used for. Seems like a good protein source and nature just gives them to us by the millions. If displayed and prepared right I would eat bugs. A lot of them are edible just ask Bear Grylls, yum.

However there are those that are intolerable and must be controlled, like mosquitoes which spread a number of diseases like Dengue Fever, Malaria, West Nile virus, just to name a few. We also have the flea, which can spread Bubonic Plague, which killed approximately half the world's population in the dark ages.

With parasites and bloodsuckers being the major pests, we need insecticides; they are necessary for the better health of our pets and for us. Just make them eco-friendly and if you are not the maker than use only the biodegradable ones "please". As with all things made and created by man, eco-friendly products should be our main concern. We are definitely a gifted race, we have the intelligence to do many awesome things, as we create and do our great deeds we must always treat the earth with respect and awe. Without her, our mother earth, there is only death, nonexistence for us and all the other living things that call this place home.

Self Control

I am sure all of you that read this will recognize it at once, "Sticks and stones will break my bones but words will never hurt me". When I was a child that was a popular saying, it is what we were all told by our parents or adults in our lives. Do not get upset when someone calls you names or teases it will not hurt you.

As I previously wrote, mine was "Wade in the water" now I am proud of that. Go ahead and tease about my name or anything else if that is what makes you feel better, it no longer hurts me in any way. Words role off my back like water roles off a ducks back, I would like to think that is what maturity and self-confidence will get you. Those people who are name callers and teasers usually have low self-esteem and lack confidence in themselves, they do these things to make themselves feel better.

I call that the bully syndrome and those of you who are adults and are still affected by the name calling in my opinion need to build on your own self-confidence and reach some level of maturity. We have been given the right to freedom of speech. That right has been abused and now some things we say are considered a crime. Santa Claus cannot even say HOHOHO any more.

Self-control is now being enforced to some degree anyway, because the old childhood saying no longer holds true, it is now "Sticks and stones will break my bones and names will also hurt me". It seems to me we need to toughen up and not be so sensitive, we are not nearly as tough as we used to be. However for those that are just cruel and do evil deeds for nothing more than to cause another pain, may you be given the chance at redemption. Perhaps you will be one of the lucky ones but that is for another to decide. All I can do is give my opinion, making a change in yourself is up to you.

If you are over weight and have health issues because of it, it is most likely the life style and habits you have been conditioned too. Self-control over your food consumption is the key to your weight problems. More water less sugar laden drinks more fruit less candies and cake and ice cream, more fish and chicken and less red meat. These small steps are a good and easy start to better health. Then do not forget exercise, a walk or run, swimming is great or you can play a sport.

It is quite simple really, it is common sense, but it takes effort and initiative to form good habits. What I see is a society that has become very lazy.

Plants

Almost everything we need to live on comes from plants. They give off oxygen and consume carbon dioxide through photosynthesis. In them are the cures for many aliments.

Plantain is a plant that is sometimes referred to as natures Band-Aid, has the ability to stick to the skin without artificial means. Used as a poultice it has the ability to draw out infection or splinters, foxtails and more. From personal experience, I was bitten by a Brown Recluse Spider three separate times in one year; it seems they had invaded my underwear drawer. Using the mixture of plantain, Charcoal and Alcohol I was able to prevent infection, draw out the poison and heal the wound, not only for myself but also for several other people that were bitten as well that same year.

Purslane is a weed to most people; it grows readily in gardens, yards, and fields' excreta. This plant is good in salads; you can pickle it or juice it. Purslane is full of beneficial uses, it is high in Omega 3, it also has large amounts of vitamin E. When made in to a tea it can be helpful in soothing the irritation of a urinary track infection.

Stinging Nettle contains chlorophyll, vitamins A, b2, C, E and K1, folic acid, histamine, acetylcholine, formic acid, acetic acid and butyric acid plus an abundance of minerals. Everyone I know hates this plant because of the irritating hairs and burning sensation when brushed up against the skin. The constituents of this plant give it medicinal value in that it acts as a diuretic, antirheumatic and blood purifier because it speeds up your metabolism. My wife and I use it to make tea along with mint and elderberries, which by the way is extremely delicious! The leftover leaves we grind up for the dogs, which seems to help relieve certain skin allergies.

Dandelion is a common weed that so many of us love to hate. What a shame since they are completely eatable and contain many medicinal characteristics. Dandelions contain tannins, glycosidic substances, inulin, bitter principles and the milky sap constituents have a beneficial effect on liver and kidney function. It can prevent gallstones and kidney stones and if present aid in their elimination. It also relives painful arthrosis caused by excessive uric acid in joints. It also contains vitamins such as C and B2, making this a very useful weed to have around. Yet everyone tries to kill it off, calling it an eyesore in his or her yard.

Wow some amazing plants, otherwise known as weeds.

This is just to mention a few of the thousands of plants that can and will help you if take the time to learn what nature has provided. Many of these plants grow in our own back yard and we have a tendency to want to poison them and destroy what nature has given us as a gift. We are just now beginning to realize organic is the way to go. If we would harvest what grows in our yards instead of poisoning them we would save money, save the earth and live healthier. .

I remember my first experience with stinging nettle very well. It is a memory I hope I never forget, for it is one of grave discomfort. It began one bright and sunny morning, hunting squirrel with my father and brother in the coulees of South Eastern Minnesota. This is a hardwood forest area where oaks, hickory and walnut trees are in abundance and so are the squirrels. These rodents of the trees or more commonly known as "Tree rats" where I come from are quite large and come in red, black and grey, I've even seen a white one. These were a common food source for our family. For all of you who have never had squirrel they are quite tasty.

Well as it turned out Mother Nature called, and wouldn't you know it, no toilet paper, no napkins, no nothing. Therefore, my father tells me to pick some soft green leaves and use that in place of toilet paper, so I did. The leaves I chose were very soft with little hairs. They looked like they would do well. I stroked the leaves taking care to be thorough, pleased with my nice soft choice of vegetation. Then all of a sudden, my buttocks started stinging, prickling burning and itching. That my friend is a sensation you really do not want to experience.

I later found out that it was a plant called Stinging Nettle and rightfully so. Well I did not tell my dad or brother for fear of being embarrassed and their laughing stock. I went through the whole day with butt burning and stinging on fire with no relief to the torture that I had inflicted upon myself. That is one plant I have never forgot and over the years I have learned a lot about, all of its benefits as well as the tortures of its bite.

Book End

Being "One With Nature" can be done in many ways, from eating the natural plants that grow in your yard to having solar roof shingles supply your electrical needs around your home. Electric autos and hybrids are all helpful, so is carpooling, using only organic based materials and pesticides, cleaners, etc. If you do not use the poisons, the manufacturers will stop making them. They will only make what people want to buy, remember if you demand only eco-friendly products, that is what manufacturers will supply. Every consumer controls at least part of what happens to our planet by what they consume. So we must change our habits if want to live on in harmony with mother earth. You know what they say, "Better late than never", my hope in writing this book is to help educate man kind to show that there is hope, a better way of living and to be "One With Nature".

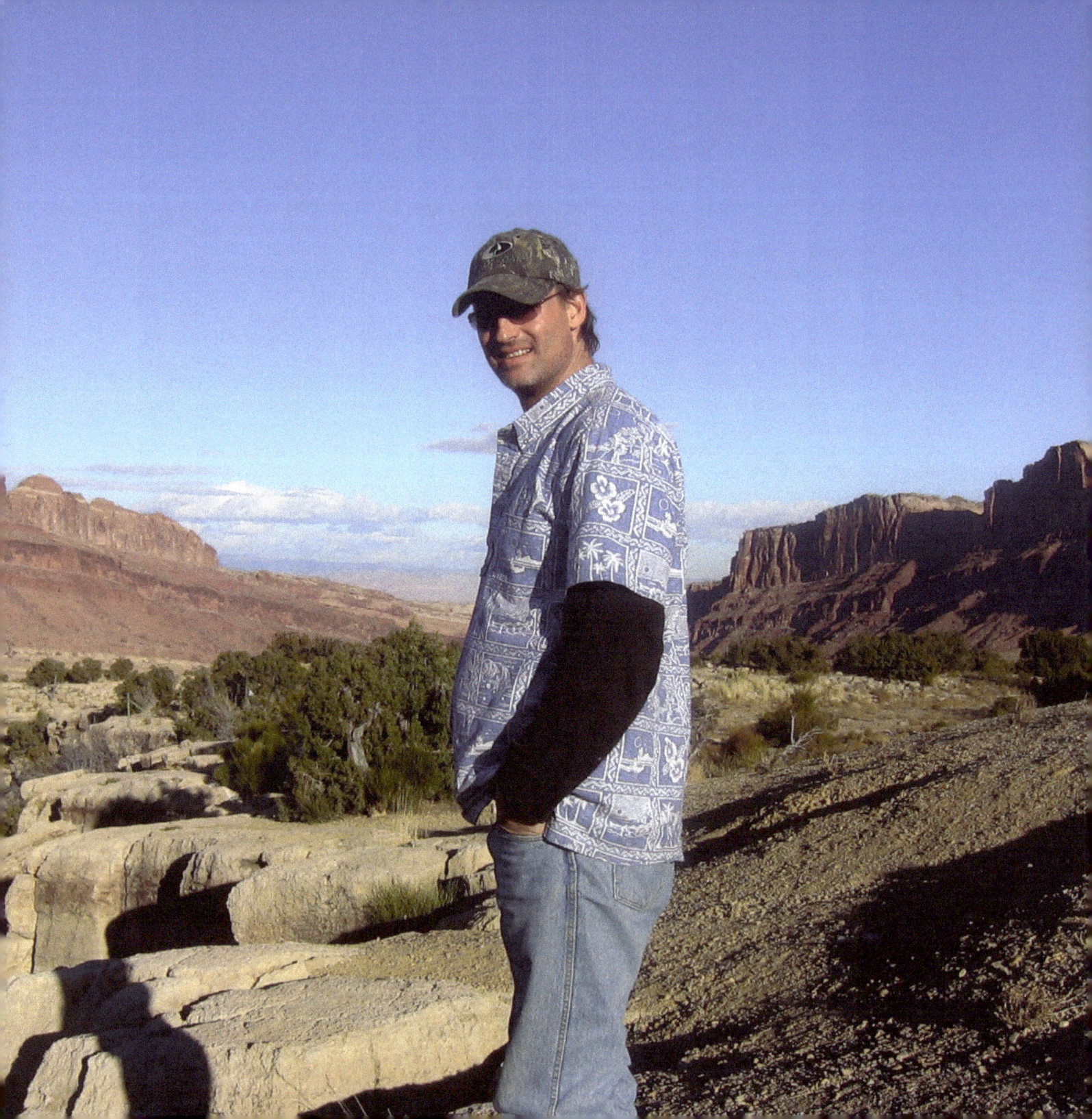

About the Author

I was born in Minnesota, one of three children in my family. I have a brother one year older and a sister that is no longer with us. I left Minnesota when I was twenty-one; from there I traveled and worked doing every thing from door to door sales, tree trimming, real estate and then construction. I got married when I was forty-eight, it took me that long to find my soul mate. Some things are worth waiting for.

www.ingramcontent.com/pod-product-compliance
Lightning Source LLC
Chambersburg PA
CBHW040544220526
45473CB00016B/3012